Clinical Neurology Made Easy

Bertha Chioma Ekeh

B, Med Pharm, MBBS, FMCP (Neuro)

Front cover image culled from
http://factsforkids.net/brain-facts-kids-top-15-mind-blowing-facts-human-brain-2/

Copyright © 2018 Bertha Chioma Ekeh

All rights reserved.

ISBN-10: 1723869440
ISBN-13: 978-1723869440

DEDICATION

I dedicate this book to the **Almighty God** for giving me everything: Life, Family, Health, Knowledge, and everything that I am today.

To my late mother Mrs. Celina Onwueyiagba Ekeh who died of complications of Stroke on January 8th 1999. Mma; I just wish I knew what I know now then. I am who I am today because of the great woman that you are.

To my late father Mr Lawrence Onuawuchi Ekeh; Renowned Educationist who taught me to teach.

To my siblings: Anie, Agatha, Loretta and Izuchi; Thank you for sharing my joys, successes, pains, tears and for believing in me.

To Emerson and Shauntae: Thank you for taking time to find us.

CONTENTS

	Acknowledgments	I
1	Introduction	1
2	History Taking	8
3	Mental System Examination	29
4	The Cranial Nerves	58
5	Motor System Examination	81
6	Sensory System Examination	109
7	Other Examinations	120
8	Examination of the Unconscious Patient	134

ACKNOWLEDGMENTS

ACKNOWLEDGMENTS

Prof Nwadiuto Akani: Department of Paediatrics, University of Port Harcourt, Nigeria
You acknowledged that Neurology is challenging and gave me the needed courage to study it. Your honesty made me the neurologist that I am today. Thank you Ma

Dr Kingsley Mayowa Okunoda:
Lecturer/ Consultant Psychiatrist. Department of Psychiatry, Univeristy of Jos, Nigeria
You asked me to write a book to make Neurology easy. Thank you for giving me the idea. I hope I succeeded in making it easy.

Dr Udeme Ekrikpo: Lecturer/ Consultant Nephrologist
Department of Internal Medicine, University of Uyo, Nigeria
You were a pillar of support and encouragement during the writing of this book. Thank you

PREFACE

When I was a medical student, I was afraid of Neurology like most medical students all over the world. It was considered a very difficult aspect of Medicine. Taking the history in neurological disorders and the neurological examination seemed like an insurmountable Herculean task. We watched our senior colleagues talking major 'stuff' above our heads. A neurology case during a clinical examination was tantamount to 'Death Sentence'. All these changed when Dr N Akani (then a senior registrar in Paediatrics) acknowledged that she was once afraid of Neurology and encouraged me to give it a little more attention. Her honesty made me to take up the challenge to study and understand Neurology also.

Having unravelled Neurology, I determined to make it easier for those coming behind me; this I have successfully done in teaching Neurology to different sets of medical students from University of Jos, University of Ibadan and now University of Uyo all in Nigeria.

My greatest joy and fulfillment comes when my students reply; **'Thank you ma, you have made it easy'.**

This book is an extension of that same passion to simplify neurology for all the Medical students, Medical Doctors and Neurology residents all over the world. In writing this book therefore, I have a much larger class. 'Clinical Neurology Made Easy' presents history taking and neurological examination in a simplified manner without compromising the knowledge. This book therefore is a reminder of the importance of a detailed methodical clinical evaluation. It is also gives assurance to doctors and neurologists in poor resource settings that the diagnosis of neurological disorders is not impossible but rather it is within reach with good clinical evaluation.

In fact this is the book I wish I had read!!!

Bertha Chioma Ekeh

PART ONE

HISTORY TAKING IN NEUROLOGY

CHAPTER 1
INTRODUCTION

1.1 Definition

History taking like in all aspects of medicine is of paramount importance in the Neurology patient. History is derived from two words (*his* and *story*). This summarizes what history entails; ***History is the patient's story.*** A skilful approach to the history is often required in all specialties in Medicine to get the essential details. In neurology, more than any other specialty, the physician is dependent upon the cooperation of the patient for a reliable history. This is especially so for a description of symptoms that are not accompanied by obvious signs of the disease. The first step is to win the patients trust, confidence and cooperation. Ability to communicate with the patient is his local language is an advantage especially in practices like mine where there are lots of uneducated patients. Patience is needed since most neurology patients have been seen by many doctors before the referral and are usually fatigued. *Attention to the patient's description of symptoms usually helps in the accurate localization of the lesion*. This localization is of paramount importance because it guides the examination, ensures relevant investigations and eventual diagnosis. Often, the history requires collaboration from a near relative or the caregiver (Informant) in some neurological disorders like seizures, dementia, loss of consciousness. The history from the patient alone is incomplete in such cases since the patient is either forgetful or was unaware or unconscious at the time of the event.

It is noteworthy that most neurological diagnosis (>90%) will be made with good clinical acumen. This is particularly thrilling for doctors practicing in poor resource settings who do not have access to most of the current equipment for investigations. Many errors therefore result from over-reliance on imaging studies, electrophysiology and laboratory tests at the expense of good history and examination.

1.2 The Biodata

The patient's personal data make one individual differ from another. They are very important in the epidemiology of diseases. Common diseases occur commonly e.g. Multiple sclerosis is more likely in a Caucasian residing in the temperate climate than in a Negro residing in the tropics. Infectious diseases are more likely in the tropics than the western world. Connective tissue and autoimmune disorders are commoner in women than in males. Neurodegenerative diseases are commoner in the older patients than in the young. It is therefore extremely important to get the biodata correctly and take it into consideration in making a clinical diagnosis.

Components of the biodata are as follows:

Name
The name is the patient's first identity and gives a lot of information. The name of the patient should

be written correctly. In a country like Nigeria with multiple ethnicities, the name of an individual identifies him with his ethnic group and possible geographic location. The name therefore may correlate with certain ethnic practices or beliefs which may enlighten the doctor on the possible etiology, or beliefs and practices that may further alter the course of the illness.

Nigerians generally enjoy titles and the proper recognition and use of the title will make the history taking easier because the patient will be more cooperative if correctly addressed. This is especially so with elderly patient when the doctor is young; failure to identify and use the correct title is considered disrespect on the part of the young doctor. Medical students are therefore taught to be mindful of these mundane but important issues that markedly affect the details of the history.

Age
The age of the patient is extremely important. Epidemiology of diseases is greatly determined by the persons age. Cerebrovascular Disease (Stroke) and neurodegenerative diseases commonly affect the elderly. Epilepsy usually starts during childhood and teenage years. Hence it commonly affects the young. In underdeveloped countries like Nigeria, the birth records were not properly kept some decades ago. For such patients, major events in the country are used to estimate the age. Commonly in Nigeria, these are: the Nigerian independence in 1960, and the Nigerian civil war (1967-1970).

Address
The patient's address is usually a reflection of the social status. The social status is essential in the etiology, epidemiology and health seeking behaviour of the patient. In addition, in many countries in sub Saharan Africa (SSA), healthcare is paid for from out of pocket expenses. The social status and available funds may determine the type of investigations and medications each patient can afford , considering that most African patients pay for healthcare from 'out of pocket'. Finally, the address is also important as regards patient's accessibility to health for those who will need physiotherapy and further follow-up.

Marital Status
The marital status of the patient gives an idea of his social life. The presence of a significant other may impact on the type of care the patient may receive especially in those with chronic disorders that will need long periods of care. This is important in countries in SSA where there are no rehabilitation centers and hospice care. Married patients have more support and care from their spouses and children.

Religion
Africans are generally very religious. These religious beliefs vary even amongst the same religion. The religious belief therefore may affect the diagnosis of the patient and may also alter the treatment.Most neurological disorders are generally considered spiritual diseases because of their

presentations. This includes cerebrovascular disorders, epilepsy, peripheral neuropathies, dementia and others. These beliefs greatly affect the health-seeking behaviours of the patients. Some Christian denominations do not accept orthodox medical treatment. It is important to find out whether the denomination is the Jehovah witnesses who do not believe in blood transfusion in order to ensure that they are treated with care and sensitivity when there is need for blood transfusion.

Race/Ethnic Group
Certain diseases are common in certain races example, Sickle Cell disease in the African Negro and Lipid storage disease in the Ashkenazi Jews. In Africa, the numerous ethnic groups have different practices that predispose them to different diseases. The belief in black magic traverses the continent. Most neurological diseases like Stroke are therefore considered a spiritual attack. This belief is common in most African cultures. Hence patients with stroke are more likely to be taken to the traditional healer or church than the hospital. This also happens in the cases of epilepsy, paraplegia and in peripheral neuropathies. Epilepsy and Dementia are particularly stigmatized in most ethnic groups in SSA. Elderly patients with Dementia are regarded as witches in some ethnic groups and hence may be victims of elder abuse. There may also be ethnic practices that predispose to certain conditions.

Occupation
Certain occupations predispose patients to certain diseases. Long distant drivers in Nigeria are predisposed to HIV/AIDS which may have neurological manifestations. Farmers who wade through murky water are predisposed to schistosomiasis which may have neurological complications. The diagnosis may also be the cause for change of profession. The patient with epilepsy and sleep disorders will be encouraged from occupations that will involve handling heavy machinery, driving or climbing.

Conclusion
The biodata defines the patient as an individual who is different from the next person in different ways. Exploring the biodata helps the doctor to establish rapport with the patient while giving the doctor information on the patient's uniqueness. In the author's practice where there are multiple ethnic groups and languages, the evaluation of the patient is much easier when the doctor speaks the same language as the patient since most persons are apprehensive of a stranger.

CHAPTER 2

THE NEUROLOGY HISTORY

2.1 The Presenting Complaint
Common symptoms of neurological disease include the following:

Headache
Seizures
Weakness
Loss of Consciousness
Memory loss
Abnormal Movements
Sensory Disturbances
Sleep Disturbances
Vertigo and Disturbances
Speech abnormalities

Headache
Headache is the commonest neurological symptom in adults: the estimate being that 98% of all adults have had a headache at one point of time or the other. In taking a history of headache, the duration and frequency are important. The duration defines an acute or chronic disease. The characteristics are those of a history of pain. The acronym *'SOCRATES'* used in taking a history of pains also applies to history taking in headache. Components are; the *site* of the pain which could be the forehead, temporal, cervical or occipital area. Temporal headaches are usually from causes within the anterior fossa while frontal headaches are either

from pathologies in the paranasal sinuses or the eyes. Occipital and cervical headaches commonly refer to lesions of the posterior fossa. The headache could be unilateral like in migraine or bilateral like in tension headache. It may be located in the temporal area as seen in temporal arteritis or around the eye like in cluster headache. The *onset* may be sudden or gradual. Headaches caused by meningitis, subarachnoid haemorrhage, migraine and cluster headaches are usually of sudden onset. Whereas those from, brain masses or space occupying lesions are of gradual onset. The *character* of the pain may be throbbing like in migraine, boring like in cluster headache or thunder-clasp like in SAH or heavy like in tension headache. The headache may *radiate* to the neck, eyes, face or teeth. Cervical pain from cervical spondylosis causes electric like shock sensations through the arms on bending the neck. Headaches may be *associated* with lacrimation and redness of the eyes. Nausea and vomiting, visual loss or scotomas may be seen in migraine. There may be associated fever and neck stiffness in meningitis or jaw claudication in temporal arteritis. There may be other associated neurological symptoms like seizures, loss of consciousness or weakness of one side of the body especially seen in brain haemorrhage. Dizziness and vertigo may be associated features in some cases. *Timing* of the headache is important. Headaches may be always present, or come on and off. Headaches that disturb sleep are worrisome. Cluster and hypnic headaches are characteristically nocturnal. This typical history is very important. Headaches from brain tumours are usually early in the morning. It is also important to note how long the headaches last.

Migraine headache lasts between 4-72 hours after which it abates on its own. Cluster headaches peak in 15-45 minutes but characteristically last about 2 hours. These primary headaches may become chronic daily headaches and hence last longer than the stipulated period. Find out whether there are ***exacerbating or relieving*** factors. Usually sleep should abate headaches therefore, it is important to ask whether the headache disturbs sleep. Headaches in raised intracranial pressure may be worsened by increased intra-abdominal pressure which is caused by coughing, micturition, lifting heavy objects. Migraine headaches may be precipitated by exertion, fatigue, poor sleep or certain foods. Some headaches are more *severe* than others. It is worthy of note that as much as 90% of headaches are benign. Hunger, anger, poor sleep, noise, fatigue, emotional upset, physical or psychological stress may all cause severe headaches with no neurological disease.

Below are features that suggest an underlying disorder (Significant Headaches):

i) Sudden-onset headache
ii) First severe headache
iii) "Worst" headache ever
iv) Vomiting that precedes headache
v) Subacute worsening over days or weeks
vi) Pain induced by bending, lifting, cough

vii) Pain that disturbs sleep or presents immediately upon awakening
viii) Known systemic illness
ix) Onset after age 55
x) Fever or unexplained systemic signs
xi) Abnormal neurologic examination
xii) Pain associated with local tenderness, e.g., region of temporal artery

These features should also be explored with direct questions while taking a history of headaches.

Seizures

Seizures are common presenting complaints in the neurology clinic. In fact, most young patients in the adult neurology clinic in SSA present with seizures. It is important to define whether there has been a seizure or not. A good history of seizure usually requires an eye witness account. History of seizure should include the description of the type whether generalized or focal. The duration of the seizure, associated loss of consciousness should be ascertained. Other important features are the history of biting of the tongue and lips, upward rolling of the eyes, faecal and urinary incontinence. The history of the post-ictal period should include associated post-ictal sleep and the duration, headaches, weakness and confusion. Is there extreme weakness of one side of the body for hours or even days (Todd's palsy)? Are there periods of absent mindedness which may indicate absence seizures? Are there periods of behavioural arrest or abnormal behaviours which are features of complex partial seizures? Take further history of the frequency of the seizure, possible precipitants, a preceding aura, premonitory or warning symptoms and previous head trauma. Does the seizure have a Jacksonian march (a gradual step-wise progression from digits upwards to the head)? In places where seizures are stigmatized like in my practice, some patients may not accept that they are having seizures.

They may give a history of frequents falls, collapse or even headaches. In such scenarios, you have to ask direct questions comprising the following features which are important in differentiating seizures (fits) between syncope (faints); the commonest and most mistaken differential.

Table 1
Differentiating between seizures and syncope

Features	Seizure	Syncope
Preceding Symptoms	Aura	Dizziness Sweating Palpitations Blackouts
Time of onset	Daytime or Night time	Daytime
Posture	Occurs in any posture	Occurs in persons in upright postures
Convulsions	Multiple jerks	Few jerks
Automatisms	May be present	Absent

Facial and buccal wounds	Present	Absent
Post Ictal Phenomenon (Headaches, lethargy. confusion)	Present	Absent
Urinary or fecal incontinence	May be present	Absent
Blood Pressure	Normal or Increased	Decreased
General examination	Cyanosis	Pallor

There are also some persons who have nocturnal seizures but no seizures in the daytime; hence they give a negative history of seizures. In these circumstances, a history of waking up from sleep with wounds in the mouth, urinary incontinence, lethargy, confusion and or headaches will suggest a seizure. Note that certain persons who give a history of the post ictal phenomenon like headache, lethargy and confusion while denying the occurrence of a seizure. Further history to determine the aetiology of the seizure will include the history of childhood illnesses, head trauma, pregnancy and birth history and family history.

Weakness

Many neurological disorders present with weakness of the limbs. The first step is to identify the site of the weakness. Does the weakness involve one side of the body, the two lower limbs, one limb, all four limbs and rarely three limbs? Is there associated weakness of the face (deviation of the mouth to one side)? Involvement of the face is usually seen in a hemispheric lesion. Ask whether the weakness was sudden or gradual in onset. Sudden weakness of one side of the body is characteristic of stroke. Are there associated or preceding features? Associated sudden speech impairment, visual disturbances, sensory disturbances and imbalance are also in keeping in stroke.

Weakness of the lower limbs may be sudden or gradual. Sudden weakness of the lower limbs is caused by trauma, anterior two third syndrome, transverse myelitis, Guillain Barre Syndrome and or Spondylolisthesis. Most other etiologies are more gradual. Compressive cord lesions are usually preceded by waist or back pains with associated disturbance of the sphincters; urinary retention or incontinence/constipation or fecal incontinence. Potts disease is a common cause of weakness of the lower limbs in the SSA. The classical presentation is that of waist and or back pains for weeks before gradual weakness of the lower limbs and eventual involvement of the sphincters and total paralysis. In motor neuropathies, myopathies and neuromuscular junction diseases the typical presentation is proximal weakness. In these cases, the muscles of the shoulder and pelvic girdles (proximal muscles) are weak hence there will be a history of difficulty in climbing the staircase, standing up and rising from a squatted or seated position. There is also difficulty in raising the arms above the head, unscrewing a light bulb, hanging clothes on a line and others. Associated features are difficulty in swallowing, drooling of saliva, slurring of speech (due to weakness of the cranial muscles). Myasthenic weakness is also characterized by fatiguability and worsened by exertion, and poor sleep. The patient is stronger after rest or sleep. There may be a history of frequent falls because the muscles of the pelvis and the thighs are the weight bearing muscles of the body. Guillain Barre Syndrome is known to cause acute ascending paralysis with mild non-definitive pains. Motor neurone disease is gradually progressive and the weakness takes years before the patient presents for care.

Loss of consciousness
Unconsciousness is a sleep like state with unawareness of self and environment and no response to external stimulus or inner need. *In essence an unconscious patient is asleep.* However, unconsciousness differs from the physiological sleep in that the individual cannot be aroused by external stimulus (bright lights, noise etc) or inner need (hunger, thirst, micturition, defecation). Loss of consciousness could be transient or continuous. Transient loss of consciousness which is characterized by spontaneous recovery is usually not of neurological origin. The commonest causes are arrhythmias and syncope. A seizure is the commonest neurological cause of transient loss of consciousness. *In fact, transient loss of consciousness with full spontaneous recovery is considered a seizure until proven otherwise.*

History of loss of consciousness will include duration of the loss of consciousness which may be of sudden onset and dramatic as seen in stroke. Unconsciousness may also be gradual having been preceded by headaches, vomiting, irrational behaviours and restlessness as seen in metabolic encephalopathies and also associated fever in acute bacterial meningitis. There may be a history of other associated features like seizures, headaches, sudden collapse, fever, neck stiffness and vertigo. A history of lack of food intake before the loss of consciousness is essential to the diagnosis of hypoglcaemia. A past medical history of Hypertension, Diabetes Mellitus, Epilepsy, HIV/AIDS or other disorders is very important in the evaluation and eventual diagnosis since the cause of the unconsciousness may a complication of these prior diagnoses. Further history should include history of previous head trauma or innocuous falls in the elderly, any medications in use and possible overdose, and alcohol intake.

Confusion

Confusion is a vague term that lacks precision. In general, it denotes the inability to think with customary speed, clarity and coherence. The history of confusion should include the duration, the preceding event, fever, headache, and seizures. Take a history of previous medical diseases like hypertension, diabetes mellitus liver and kidney pathologies. A patient with receptive aphasia is usually said to be confused given that the relatives are unable to understand him/her. In the elderly;

some diseases have an atypical presentation hence, myocardial infarction and infections like urinary tract and chest infections may present with confusion. *Note that a confused elderly patient is usually not a psychiatric patient but a neurological patient.* Common causes of confusion in the elderly include sepsis, hypertensive encephalopathy, Hyperglycaemic Hyperosmolar States and Uraemia.

Abnormal movements

Involuntary movements are usually embarrassing to the patients especially when the face is involved. The duration of these movements should be ascertained; persons with tremors present after months or years while those with hemiballismus and myoclonus present within hours or days. The onset of the abnormal movements is an important part of the history. Ask whether the movements were of sudden or gradual onset. *Abnormal violent movements (mainly unilateral) that start suddenly are in keeping with hemiballismus.* Most of the other movements are more gradual in onset. The movements may be rhythmical or arrhythmical. Tremors are rhythmical while all the others are arrhythmical. Ask whether the movements are unilateral or bilateral? Tremors in Parkinson disease classically start from one side of the body and later involve the other side while benign essential tremors involve both aspects of the body from the onset. Hemiballismus is usually unilateral but may be bilateral (ballismus) while chorea is typically bilateral but may be unilateral (hemichorea).

Which parts of the body are involved in the movement? Chorea classically involves the lower limbs while hemiballismus affects the upper limb. Tremors and dystonias may involve the head, tongue and the lips while head tremors are not seen in Parkinson disease. *In fact head and neck tremors are unknown in Parkinson disease; presencee of head and neck tremors all but rules out Parkinson disease.* Also ask whether the movements are fast or slow? Athetosis and dystonia are slow while chorea, tics

Myoclonus and hemiballismus are fast. Note that tics can be suppressed by voluntary control. Tremors are the commonest abnormal movements. They are characteristically rhythmical that is two-way movements: flexion- extension, pronation – supination, left- right, up-down, open and close. Flexion-extension tremor of the head (Titubation) is a feature of cerebellar disorder. Tremors could be at rest as seen in Parkinson disease or intention tremors like in cerebellar diseases or postural like in thyrotoxicosis. Do the movements disappear during sleep? *Movement disorders usually disappear in sleep while sleep related movement disorders appear during sleep.* Drug induced movement disorders are common and present acutely after days or weeks of ingestion of the medications. Note that Parkinson disease is not an acute disease. A history of acute symptoms suggestive of Parkinson disease will be either drug or toxin induced. Commonest medications that cause Parkinsonian symptoms are the neuroleptics and Metoclopromide.

Sensory disturbances
Sensory disturbances could present in a variety of ways and are usually troubling to the patient because of the abnormal feelings. There may be loss of feeling, numbness or a feeling of deadness. These are referred to as negative symptoms. The positive symptoms are pins and needles sensation, burning sensation, pains. Important aspects of the history include the duration. Is it acute, sub-acute or chronic? What is the part of the body involved? Sensory disturbance on one side of the body is in keeping with lacunar stroke or seizures. Whereas the sensory disturbance will be continuous, the sensory seizure will be paroxysmal. Occasionally, the sensory seizure may have a Jacksonian march. The feet and hands are typically involved in distal symmetrical polyneuropathies because of the dying back phenomenon. Entrapment neuropathies have a limited representation affecting few fingers. Plexopathies affect the area of innervations of the plexus. Are the symptoms worse at night? Are there any variations with movement, sleep, walking or rest?

Dizziness/Vertigo
Dizziness actually covers so many complaints from vague feelings of unsteadiness, faint or light headedness which are felt in panic and anxiety states. Vertigo defines an illusion of movement. Patients complain of a sensation of rotation, falling

oscillating or tipping. The patient will feel that he or the environment is moving when they are not. They may feel that the bed they are lying on is turning or that the car is somersaulting. One of the author's patient felt that the wall was growing upwards. There may be a history of rotating objects or movement of self or the objects in the environment. Is the vertigo of sudden or gradual onset? Sudden onset vertigo may be seen in cerebellar stroke, vertiginous seizures or vestibular neuronitis. Is the vertigo positional or it occurs irrespective of the position? Common causes of brief dizziness (seconds) include benign paroxysmal positional vertigo (BPPV) and orthostatic hypotension, both of which typically are provoked by changes in head and body position. Attacks of vestibular migraine and Meniere's disease often last hours.

When episodes are in minutes, transient ischemic attacks of the posterior circulation should be considered, although migraine and a number of other causes are also possible. Vertigo on standing up from a supine position is in keeping with Benign Paroxysmal Positional Vertigo (BPPV) whereas seizures and sensory stroke will cause vertigo in any position. There may be a history of falls. If there are falls, find out whether patient falls to a side. Is there, vomiting, mild imbalance, hearing loss or ringing sensation in the ear which may be feature of peripheral vertigo? In central vertigo, the imbalance is so severe that the patient may not be able to walk. This continous vertigo is classically seen in cerebeallar stroke.

Memory loss/forgetfulness

Forgetfulness is another important and increasingly common symptom of neurological patients. It is important to know the duration and course of the forgetfulness. In Alzheimer's disease, there is an insidious onset and gradual progression of forgetfulness. The history of forgetfulness has been there for years before presentation. Characteristically, the relatives find it difficult to define the time the forgetfulness actually started. In contrast, in multi-infarct dementia, there are dramatic episodes of forgetfulness. In fact astute caregivers can give dates of distinct sudden episodes. What does the patient forget? Does he forget his personal items like tooth brush, comb, wristwatch, spectacles and items of clothing. Can he/she match his clothes properly? Can he recognize and call names of close relatives correctly? The information the patient forgets should be ascertained. Is he able to follow conversation and relay messages? Does the patient wander away and is unable to find his way home? Can he find his way around in a familiar environment? Is the patient able to handle money; does he still know the purchasing power of a certain amount of money? Can he carry out his banking transactions? Is there personality or behavioural changes from his norm? Has the patient become difficult to relate with?

Difficulty in speaking
Difficulty in speaking is another common presentation in the neurology clinic. Some of the patients are unable to say a word or make themselves to be understood. In such cases, a reliable informant is needed to give the history. Was

the difficulty in speaking sudden or gradual in onset? Sudden difficulty in speaking or inability to speak is in keeping with Stroke. The history should explore whether the abnormality is in poor expression or understanding of spoken speech. Patients with receptive aphasia are unable to comprehend speech. They are usually thought to be confused because they can neither understand themselves nor others. The author had such a patient who as a nursing mother didn't pick up her crying baby till concerned neighbours rushed in and found her unable to speak or understand speech. Her eventual diagnosis was stroke. If the patient can understand and comprehend speech, then is he able to understand but cannot express him. History should include the loudness of speech, proper articulation of words and clarity of the speech. Patients with speech disorders may be labeled as confused since they are often unable to communicate well.

2.2 Past Medical History

The past medical history is of paramount importance. A previous diagnosis of hypertension, diabetes mellitus, sickle cell disease, epilepsy, a malignancy, previous stroke or a cardiac disease may be significant. Headache and seizures in a patient with a previous diagnosis of hypertension may be a harbinger of hypertensive encephalopathy or the more sinister haemorrhagic stroke. In a patient with altered consciousness, the history of a previous innocuous head trauma in the elderly may be a pointer to sub acute subdural haematoma. The history of trauma with an open wound would precede the lock jaw and spasms points to a diagnosis of tetanus. The patient with a cerebral abscess will have a previous history of penetrating head trauma, sinusitis, otitis media or pneumonia. Certain malignancies have neurological disorders as para neoplastic features. Previous diagnosis of HIV/AIDS may help in making a diagnosis of Progressive multifocal leucoencephalopathy in a person with seizures, headaches and or gradual weakness of one side of the body. A history of recurrent abortions may suggest antiphospholipid syndrome in a young woman with Stroke.

2.3 Obstetrics and Gynaecology History

All women should have this history explored. The menarche, last menstrual period and previous pregnancies are important. Ask for a history of recurrent abortions which may be as a result of antiphospholipid syndrome. History of oral contraceptives may be related to the headaches. In a patient with sensory disturbance, the previous history of large or malformed babies is in keeping with Diabetes Mellitus. A patient with recurrent abortions and headache or sensory disturbance may have an eventual diagnosis of Systemic Lupus Erythemathosus (SLE). A woman of child bearing age with bleeding par vaginaum, weight loss and headache may have choriocarcinoma.

2.4 Pregnancy and Birth History

This history is important in young patients with neurological disease like epilepsy, cerebral palsy and mental retardation. Ask for a history of medical illnesses during pregnancy. Febrile illnesses are particularly important in Nigeria. History of prolonged labour, birth injuries and birth asphyxia are important. Finally the history of neonatal illnesses like Jaundice and sepsis should be taken.

2.5 Drug History
This includes the prescribed drugs used for medical illnesses. These may have neurological side effects. The calcium channel antagonists cause headaches. Neuroleptics are common causes of abnormal movements. Numerous drugs cause peripheral neuropathies. Certain drugs have been associated with Parkinson disease. Ask for a history of over the counter medications. Nigerians also use a lot of traditional herbs which contain unknown substances. These practices are seen in all the ethnic groups and even in all educational levels and social classes. Many diseases therefore have been altered before the patient arrives in the hospital.

2.6 Family and Social History
In medical diseases, the family of origin of the patient may have history of a similar disease like in the case of stroke, epilepsy, familial tremors and Neurofibromatosis. The family's response to the patient's illness may alter the cause of the disease. This is especially so in diseases with a social stigma like epilepsy.

Alcohol History

Take a history of significant alcohol intake which is 21 or more units/week for men and 14 or more units for women. In Nigeria where the author practices, the most popular type of alcohol is beer. A bottle of beer contains approximately 5.5% alcohol.

Each bottleof beer has a volume of 60cl/600mls

In 100mls of beer, there is 5g of alcohol and therefore 33g (6x5.5) of Alcohol in the 600mls.

1 unit of alcohol is equivalent to 8g

Number of units in each bottle of beer, will be

33 ÷ 8 =4.125 units of Alcohol

Significant alcohol intake in men is 21units.

No of bottles of beer that make 21 units = (21 ÷ 4.12) =5.09 bottles

Hence more than 6 bottles of Nigerian beer/week is significant alcohol intake for men.

In women, significant Alcohol intake is > 14 units/week

Number of bottles that make 14 units of Alcohol is (14 ÷ 4.125) = 3.39 bottles

Hence, more than 4 bottles of Nigerian beer /week is significant Alcohol intake for women. Significant alcohol consumption is a risk factor for Stroke, dementia, peripheral neuropathies. It is also associated with Wernicke- Korsakoff's psychosis. Noteworthy is the fact that persons with significant alcohol consumption have frequent falls and are predisposed to acute subdural haematoma. Alcohol is also a precipitating factor for seizures in persons with Epilepsy.

Smoking

The history of cigarette smoking is important. Cigarette smoking is a recognized risk factor for Stroke. The number of pack years is calculated as

No of cigarettes /no of sticks in the pack (20) x no of years smoked. Significant smoking is 10 pack years. Some Nigerians also take the local snuff which also contains a lot of Nicotine.

History of recreational drugs (Cocaine, Heroine) should be taken especially in the young. These may cause haemorrhagic stroke in the young adult. Patients with drug withdrawal also present with neurological features.

2.7 Role of Informants in History Taking

The role of informants cannot be over emphasized in history taking. This is more so in neurological disorders. Often times, like in cases of loss of consciousness form any cause, the patient is unable to contribute to the information since he is unconscious.

The doctor will have to rely on the informant. In other cases like dementia where the patient is forgetful, additional history should be taken from informant (usually the spouse, children and siblings).

These are able to give information on the patient's pre-morbid personality. They also help to confirm the information the patient is given during examination of memory and intellect. Informants are also needed in cases of sleep, seizure disorders and in patients with mental sub-normality.

It is extremely important to always take the history from a reliable informant. In my practice, many patients who are uneducated and non proficient in English language are brought to the hospital by their more learned children or relatives who reside in the city. These relatives (usually the ones that speak English) give the history based on their own impressions. These informants are usually unreliable since they do not reside with the patient. The elderly spouse or uneducated caregiver is the more reliable informant in such a scenario.

2.8 Conclusion

Medicine is a science and also an art: the fine art of human relationship. History taking is essential in the evaluation of neurological disorders and eventual diagnosis. A good history is more than half of the neurological diagnosis. Certain diagnosis like epilepsy, primary headaches, Parkinson disease etc can be made on history alone. Emphasis on the quality of the history is a cardinal part of the diagnosis. The art history taking is almost a forgotten tool especially in the developed world where a lot of special diagnostic procedures abound. There is therefore an unwholesome dependence on these diagnostic procedures which should not to be so.

PART TWO

EXAMINATION OF THE NERVOUS SYSTEM

CHAPTER 3

EXAMINATION OF THE HIGHER CORTICAL FUNCTIONS

3.1 Introduction

Generations of medical students including the author have been afraid of neurological examination and rightly so. This is because the central nervous system is the most complicated and difficult system to examine. In most cases the CNS examination is usually not carried out fully for that will be a test of tolerance and endurance for the patient. More often than not, an abridged version of the examination is all that is done. Occasionally, there is a detailed examination of one aspect of the CNS examination depending on the presenting complaint. Of utmost importance in the examination is a methodological approach. The neurologic examination begins with observation of the patient while he walks into the consulting room. The gait of the patient can be observed at this time. Certain signs can be noted while the history is being obtained. These may include the patients affect, his facial expression and even the speech. The patient's accurate, coherent accounts of events give a good assessment of the higher cortical functions. The physician should be observant as the diagnosis could be made by careful observation. One common error is to think lightly of inconsistencies in the history and inaccuracies in dates, symptoms and of the events only to discover later that these flaws in memory are essential features of the ailment. Patience, attention and concentration are the watchword.

3.2 Instruments for the examination
Besides the patient, the following items are needed for a thorough neurological examination:
Examination couch
Stethoscope
Pen torch
Tuning fork
Pins
Cotton wool
Test tubes with hot and cold water for thermal testing
Test tube with coffee for testing of smell
Two point discriminator
Patellar hammer
Ophthalmoscope
Visual acuity card
Tongue blades/ wooden spatula
Measuring tape

3.3 General Examination

In the CNS like in all other systems, a general examination cannot be overemphasized. There may also be important pointers in other systems. Of particular importance are the following:
Examination of the patient starts from the foot of the bed. Features like obesity, height, symmetry and

amputated limbs are noted from the foot of the bed. Is there a craniotomy scar or tortuous non-pulsatile temporal artery? Look for scoliosis, kyphosis or lordosis which could be a cause of cord compression? Bull neck may be a feature of Arnold-Chiari malformation.

The facial expression is very informative in the neurology patient. In Parkinson disease, the face is oily (seborrhoea) and expressionless. There is associated staring known as *'Stelwag sign'*. This is caused by the reduced frequency of blinking as a result of the bradykinesia. Stelwag sign is also a feature of thyrotoxicosis as a result of the lid retraction. Facial asymmetry is seen in patients with facial nerve palsy like Stroke or Bell's palsy. In Myasthenia gravis, the smile is a snarl. Tetanus patients have trismus and are unable to open their mouths. The dental gap is also markedly reduced.

Others obvious signs on general examination include herpes zoster ophthalmicus, sunset eyes seen in vertical gaze palsy. Dysmorphic features like low set ears, wide palpebral fissures are seen in Down's, Turner's, Noonan's syndromes. The classical butterfly rash and alopecia in a patient with severe pains of their feet and inability to walk are features suggestive of SLE. Gingival hypertrophy may be a feature of Phenytoin use. Is the person drooling saliva?

Examination of the skin may reveal lesions like café au lait patches, neuromas, fibromas, ash leaf nodules, Shagreen patches and other skin lesions. A neuro cutaneous lesion like neurofibromatosis or tuberous sclerosis may be the diagnosis in a young patient with skin lesions, seizures and mental sub normality. There may also be lesions suggestive of meningococcaemia. Pallor, jaundice, cyanosis, edema and lymphadenopathy are features of systemic disorders like infectious diseases, liver diseases or malignancies. Proptosis in a patient with tremors and headaches is in keeping with thyrotoxicosis. Hence it is always wise to carefully observe and do a general examination from the foot of the bed.

Complicated as the examination of the central nervous system is, errors and serious omissions are avoided if the examination is carried out in an orderly manner. The examination findings are also reported in the same order. In practice however, most doctors examine the particular aspect of the CNS involved having taking a history. The order of the neurological examination is as follows:

3.4 Mental/Higher Cortical Functions

The mental state is assessed very early in the examination. This may be limited to a subjective assessment of personality, memory and intelligence formed during the history taking. A patient who gives a coherent, detailed and intelligible history will not need another mental state examination. This is because the assessment has been done during the history taking.

3.41 Appearance, Behaviour and Communication

The patient's general appearance and bearing of the patient is very important. Note whether the patient is well kept or malnourished and neglected. Being dishevelled, neglected and malnourished may be an indicator of a chronic disease, alcoholism or intravenous drug abuse. If the patient is neat and well nourished, then either the disease is more acute or the patient is well catered for. Is he or she wearing mismatched clothes? This could be a feature of Dementia when procedural memory is impaired.

The patient may be agitated, disturbed or restless which is seen in acute confusional states usually from metabolic or septic encephalopathy. Note whether the person is apathetic and disinterested in his environment as seen in persons with depression or subcortical dementias. The patient may be well groomed or unkempt. Is the patient taciturn or talkative? Can he express himself or even understand speech both his and other people? Does the patient have flight of ideas or over inclusiveness? The patient's educational level and occupation also give an idea of his intellect and degree of enlightenment.

3.42 Consciousness

Consciousness is the first parameter to be examined. This is because the patient's level of consciousness determines how far and what parameters of the nervous system will be examined. There are many parts of neurological examinations that cannot be performed in the unconscious patient since the patient's cooperation is needed in most cases. A conscious patient is usually obvious.

Prior to this time, consciousness was assessed as stupor, semi coma, coma and deep coma. These terms however are vague, subjective and difficult to reproduce amongst different examiners.

In 1974, Teasdale and Jennett in Glasgow developed a system for assessment of the Conscious level. This is known as the Glasgow coma score (GCS). The GCS is widely used all over the world to assess level of consciousness. The scores are reproducible irrespective of the observer. It is objective and also has prognostication ability. The Glasgow coma scale can be carried out just as reliably by paramedics, nurses and clinicians.

Table 2: Glasgow Coma Scale

Eye Opening	Verbal Response	Motor Response
Spontaneous 4	Oriented 5	Obeys Command 6
To Call 3	Confused 4	Localizes Pain 5
To Pain 2	Inappropriate 3	Withdraws to pain 4
None 1	Incomprehensible 2	Abnormal Flexion 3
	None 1	Abnormal Extension 2
		None 1

Persons with abnormal extension usually have decerebrate posturing as well. During examination, there may be varied motor response. Pressure on the supraorbital area may produce extension response while similar pressure on the finger nail may produce flexion. One arm may localize pain while the other may flex. When this type of variability occurs, the better response is recorded because it correlates better with final outcome.

Persons with hemiparesis will be noted to have asymmetric limb response. Some writers suggest only the use of the arm response for conscious level assessment since the leg response to pain is less consistent. In addition, some of the movements may be produced from the spinal origin than from the cerebral cortex.

The best score in the GCS is 15 and the lowest is 3 representing 'None' in all the categories. Patients with a score of 8 and above have good prognosis.

The GCS however has a few draw backs as follows: Patients with aphasia and quadriplegia are scored lower than their real score. This is because the aphasia will be mistaken for poor verbal response and in the same vein; quadriplegia is also mistaken for poor motor response. Patients with a tracheotomy tube who are unable to speak are scored as number T (8T or 6T) taking into cognizance that the tracheostomy tube may be the reason the patient is unable to vocalize. In addition, some of the patients may have their eyes open and staring into space mimicking spontaneous eye opening. For such patients, the examiner should threaten the eye with the finger and if the patient blinks, the score is 4 and if such a patient does not blink, then the score is 1. The blink is a brainstem reflex and the ability to blink indicates that the brain stem is intact hence the score of 4. The inability to blink indicates that there is the brain stem is damaged.

3.43 Orientation

The patient's orientation is examined in ***time, place and person***. Disorientation is important in organic brain diseases whether chronic or acute. There are five parameters in the assessment of orientation in time. These are; the time of the day, day of the week then the date which comprises day, month and year. In essence, the patient should know that:

Today is Thursday 9th of November 2017. The time now is about 9 AM. For patients with long stay in the hospital one day eventually looks much like the other and they may not be able to know the difference therefore, the day of the week may not be very significant.

Orientation in place also comprises five parameters. These are the ward, clinic or hospital, street, city and state or country and even the bed number for those on for those on admission. Patients who are oriented in place know whether they are in the hospital, at home, market or at work. If they are in the hospital, they know which ward or clinic they are in. They should also know which hospital and in which part of the town or town the hospital is in. It is important to ask patients who have moved from another town, state or country where they are currently. Orientation in patient is assessed by the patient's personal information like name, address, and the names of spouse, children and close relatives. If the patient is there with a caregiver, ask him the name and his relationship with the person. He may call his wife his sister and call her his sister or daughter's name. Some patients with dementia may use many words to describe instead of just calling the name e.g.; one of patient's said *'that is the man I live with who is the father of my children'* instead of *'my husband'*.

3.44 Memory

Memory comprises; the ability to grasp and retain new information. It requires processing, registration and recall. It is modality- specific and related to auditory, visual, sensory or olfactory. It may be related to abstract or internalized experience. In assessment of memory, there should be consideration of the patient's educational status, degree of enlightenment and personal interest. Asking an eighty year old uneducated woman the winner of 2014 FIFA world cup will be inappropriate if she has no interest in football/soccer. Personal issues relating to her marriage, children and occupation will be more appropriate because of her personal interest.

Memory can be classified in many different ways. Classification of memory according to Duration however is the commonest classification. It is the one usually assessed in most neurology clinics.

The classification is as follows:

- Sensory Memory
-- Short term/ Immediate Memory
--- Recent/ Secondary Memory
---- Long term memory

Short term /Immediate Memory

Short term memory is the memory for events of few seconds or minutes past. It has limited capacity of 7 $\pm$ 2 numbers. To examine the short term memory, ask the patient can to say a name and then address and repeat it 5 minutes later. It can also be tested by asking the patient to repeat a sentence. Repeating a sequence of digits (Digit span) is another method. The numbers are increased one at a time as the patient repeats e.g. say after me 342, he replies 342 then 2157 and he replies 2157 then continually increase the digits, 43528, 8563247, 249803. Most people should be able to repeat seven digits forward and five digits backwards. Note that chunking increases this limited capacity e.g. 0025-6742-9812-0534.This number which has a total of 16 digits has been split into chunks of 4 and memorized 4 at a time. In this manner, it is easy to commit 16 digits to memory.

Short term memory is particularly impaired in Wernicke-Korsakoff's syndrome and in some patients with Alzheimer dementia.

Recent Memory/ Secondary memory

In chronic organic brain disorders, memory for recent events is diminished. The degree to which recent memory is lost is an index of the severity of organic brain disorder. You can test the recent memory by asking about recent television programmes like events in a popular soap opera, the last meal or details of recent major events in the community, city or country. This could be politics, natural disasters or sports. A person's accurate description of his illness during history taking is also a good test for recent memory.

Long term Memory

Long term memory is tested by asking the patient to recall events occurring at least five years earlier. This may include the names of past presidents of his country, major events in the country, state or town like elections, tragedies sporting events etc. Asking family accounts, personal issues and interests (marriages, births, deaths in the family, patient's education, and jobs businesses) usually give better results and can be assessed while taking the history. The patient's accurate account of the history especially past medical history and coherence is a good assessment of his mental status. The long term memory is relatively resistant to the effects of neurological and psychiatric diseases hence patients with memory impairment may not remember very recent events but recall events that took places decades earlier with astounding clarity. The first name is everybody's earliest memory and is never lost. All neurological and psychiatric patients can speak still remember their first names.

Long term Memory is further classified according to the content
Declarative (Explicit) and Procedural (Implicit). Declarative memory is explicit and needs to be retrieved.

Declarative memory is further subdivided into two:
Episodic
Semantic

Episodic memory is defined as memory in time and space. Episodic memory answers all the questions that start with; When? Who? Where? How? What? and Which? What is her name? Who is the Governor of your state? How many students were in the class? Episodic memory fades after a while in all normal persons. However, it can be reinforced by personal interest, novel, pleasant and traumatic experiences. Hence somebody may easily remember the name of a stranger because it is her brother's name. Alzheimer's disease causes early loss of the episodic memory.

Semantic memory is the type of declarative memory. It comprises all the unchanging facts, principles, associations and laws. Unchanging facts like the days of the week, months of the years, countries and their capitals constitute the semantic memory. Unchanging principles like the physical attributes, colour of skin belong to a particular race also constitutes the semantic memory. In some cases, the semantic memory may also be episodic e.g. who was the president of the country in the year

2012? It answers the question that starts with 'Who?' (Episodic) and it is also an unchanging fact (Semantic).

Procedural or implicit memory

The procedural memory comprises all acquired skills which have become innate and do not need retrieval. All skills acquired (taking a bath, cleaning, dressing, driving, sewing, cooking, surgical skills) belong to the procedural memory. They are performed with ease without conscious retrieval. Alzheimer's disease markedly affects the procedural memory such that the individual is unable to carry out procedures he has done with ease for many years. He may not remember the ingredients of an everyday dish. One of the author's patients was reported to have come out of the bathroom without rinsing off the soap during a bath

Visual and Auditory memory

Visual and auditory memory are actually poorly understood aspects of memory. The visual memory may be stronger than the auditory memory and vice versa. The author has a great auditory memory but a very poor visual memory.

Visual memory can be tested by giving the patient a picture and finding out how many objects he noticed in the picture. The person with a poor visual memory will not see some of the objects. This test can also indicate other lesions like hemineglect or Simultagnosia. Persons with hemineglect will see only objects on one side while those with Simultagnosia may see only the small objects and not see the larger ones or vice versa. They are unable to see all the objects simultaneously.

Auditory memory is tested by asking the patient to repeat a previously spoken message. All the answers to the specific questions on memory should be recorded verbatim.

3.45 Speech

Speech disorders are classified into:

Dysphasias; these are the disorders of structure and organization of language.

Dysarthrias: these are the defects of articulation and enunciation of speech.

Dysphonias: these are the disorders of phonation.

The first step in the analysis of speech is to differentiate between these different disorders. The assessment must be broad enough to detect subtle disorders of language. Each component of language should be tested individually and thoroughly.

Assessment of Dysphasia

Dysphasia is the disorder of the structure and organization of language. Aphasia in the severe form and commonly used term. Dysphasia is best assessed by listening to the spontaneous speech. The first step to ensure that the patient's hearing is adequate. Fluency is best examined by listening to everyday conversation. Important aspects are as follows; the number of words spoken, ability to initiate speech, word-finding pauses, hesitations or circumlocutions, articulatory agility, and prosody.

Ideally, the letter-fluency task is used to examine ability to generate words beginning with particular letters, as many as possible in 1 minute.

Often the letters *F, A,* or *S* are used. The production of fewer than 8 words beginning with the letter *F* in 1 minute, excluding proper names and their derivatives, is abnormal. Abnormality signifies frontal dysfunction, and aphasia may or may not be present. The letter –fluency test however has a bias and is best used when the doctor and patient speak the same language hence the test is not feasible in my practice where there are many ethnic groups who speak many different languages. Therefore, assessing the speech in a patient who speaks a different language is challenging but can be done through an interpreter.

In Broca's /expressive aphasia, speech is sparse and non-fluent (10 to 15 words per minute as compared with the normal 100 to 115 words per minute) . Moreover, the speech consists of mainly of nouns, transitive verbs, or important adjectives; phrase length is abbreviated and many of the small words (articles, prepositions, conjunctions) are omitted, giving the speech a telegraphic character (non fluent aphasia).

In Wernicke's or receptive aphasia however the patient speaks fluently, gestures freely, and appears strangely unaware of his deficit. Speech is produced mostly without effort (fluent aphasia).

Despite the fluency and normal prosody, the patient's speech is remarkably devoid of meaning.

The patient therefore appears to be confused.

Naming
The naming test should include a variety of objects and not just 1 or 2 personal items or pieces of clothing the examiner happens to have at hand. Realistic bedside evaluation might include 6-8 items. Items should be always be familiar everyday items like cell phones, glass case, wallet, handkerchiefs, umbrellas, combs, keys etc. Patients with anomia are unable to name these items. They can however mime the actions for which the item is used e.g., the patient given a comb or pen may attempt to comb the hair or write instead of uttering 'comb or pen' respectively.

Repetition
Speech repetition is a useful test in the assessment of dysphasias. Abnormal repetition is the hallmark of the perisylvian aphasias (the commoner type of dysphasia which originates from the usual perisylvian area of the left hemisphere). Repetition is usually preserved in the transcortical aphasias (rarer type of dysphasia which originates from the temporal and parietal cortex like the angular gyrus). Repetition should be tested for individual words, simple sentences, and complex sentences. Patients who cannot orally repeat items should be given an opportunity to copy a sentence.

Comprehension
In assessing comprehension, you can ask the patient to perform 1- and 2-part commands is a

proven way. The questions should be asked without any cues or gesticulations and see whether he understands you e.g., 'touch your right ear with your left hand'.

Reading and writing
Reading is best assessed by asking the patient to obey a simple written command for example 'Close your eyes'. Thereafter, ask the patient to write his or her name. You can also ask the patient to write his address or a complete sentence. Reading and writing are however are difficult to assess in the uneducated patients that are usually seen in the author's practice.

Dysarthria and Dysphonia
These are disorders of articulation and phonation. They are usually assessed together. There are four main types of dysarthria. Ask the patient to pronounce some words. *All types of dysarthria affect the articulation of consonants causing the slurring of speech.* In severe cases, vowels may also be distorted.

There are different types of dysarthria as follows:

Spastic dysarthria: In spastic dysarthria, the voice quality is harsh and may be strained or strangled. The person speaks as though there is increased airflow through the nose (hyper nasality) with occasional bouts of loudness. The range of movement, tongue strength and the rate of speech are reduced in fact, the tongue feels as though it is glued to the floor of the mouth.

Hyperkinetic dysarthria: The predominant symptoms are associated with involuntary movements. The voice quality is also harsh, shaky with occasional stoppages when associated with dystonias. Hyper nasality is also common. There are usually superimposed involuntary movements in speaking voluntarily. These are commonly seen in movement disorders.

Hypokinetic dysarthria: This is mainly associated with Parkinson disease. The speech is low volume and hoarseness is common (bradyphrenia). There may be monopitch, monolalia and hyper nasality.

Ataxic dysarthria: This is due to disorders of the cerebellum. The voice quality may be harsh and the loudness varies excessively to a degree that it may become explosive because of the increased effort. Hyper nasality is not common but may occur. The patients seem to place equal and excessive stress on all syllabi spoken (*scanning or staccato speech*) and the speech is usually slurred.

Flaccid dysarthria: This type of dysarthria results from damage to the lower motor neurones involved in speech. The voice is harsh and low if one vocal cord is paralyzed. In bilateral paralysis in abducted position, the voice will be breathy and inspiratory stridor may be noted. *Note that bilateral paralysis in adducted position would constitute a medical emergency since the airway will be cut off.* The person may have monopitch and monoloudness. Over time the affected muscles will atrophy.

3.46 Intelligence

Intelligence is one of the most important objectives of the interview. The National Adult Reading Test (NART) could be used since reading ability correlates closely with intelligence in the absence of other abnormalities. Make enquiries about whether the patient can read and write. You should also assess the ability to solve simple mathematical problems.

These tests do not apply in the uneducated and are rarely used in my practice. Some neurologists have made simpler adaptations that may be used.

3.47 Attention and Concentration

These are considered part of intellectual assessment by most neurologists. The tests used include the following:

Serial 7 tests: The patient is asked to subtract 7 from 100, then subtract 7 again from the result and subtract again. The correct response should go this way. 100-7 =93, 93-7=86, 86-7=79, 79-7=72 and 72-7=65.

Persons with deficits are unable to subtract each step correctly. Serial 3 can be used for people who do not have a high level of education. That will be 30-3=27, 27-3=24, 24-3=21, 21-3=18, and 18-3=15.

Trail making tests

In the trail making test, numbers 1-20 are written in a haphazard manner and the patient is asked to join the numbers serially. The period is timed. Ideally, most patients should complete the trail within 45 -

60 seconds. A period between 1-2 minutes may be pardoned for patients with a low level of education. On one occasion, a patient who was a retired accountant took about 11 minutes to complete the trail showing marked derangement. Other ways used are spelling words backwards e.g.'WORLD' and recounting the months of the year or days of the week backwards.

3.48 Judgment
Judgment is assessed by asking some questions. What will you do if you smell burning food? What will you do when you see the tap running with no receptacle? What will you do if you notice a young child crossing a busy road all alone? There will be a confused reply in patients with dementia.

3.49 Insight
The patient's insight is tested by asking the patient to interpret the meaning of simple proverbs. In most Nigerian languages, proverbs and idioms are commonly used in speeches. You can also ask him the lesson he learnt after telling him a story.

The tests of the higher cortical functions are usually abbreviated and assessed with a battery of tools. These include:
The Mini Mental State Examination (MMSE)
Montreal Cognitive Assessment (MoCA)
The General Practitioner Assessment of Cognition (GPCOG)
The Six-item Cognitive Impairment Test (6CIT)

Informant Questionnaire on Cognitive Decline in the Elderly (IQCODE).
Abbreviated Mental Test (AMT)

Of these, the MMSE is the most popular and has been widely used and validated in many studies. The MMSE however is noted to have a bias for the educated. Despite this mild limitation; it remains the most commonly used mental state examination test for most neurological examinations.

The Mini-Mental Status Examination (MMSE)

Orientation
  Time/day/date/month/year   5
  Hospital/ward/town/state/country   5
Registration
  Identify 3 objects by name   3
Attention and Calculation
  Serial 7 tests (100 minus 7 in 5 places)   5
Recall
  Recall the earlier three objects   3
Language
  Name pencil and watch   2
  Repeat "No ifs, ands, or buts"   1
  Follow a 3 step command   3
  Write "Close your eyes" and ask patient to obey the command   1
  Ask patient to write a sentence   1
  Ask patient to copy a design (interlocking pentagons)   1

This is the standard tool of evaluation.
The total possible score is 30

A score of more than 24 is normal
A score of less than 24 suggests dementia

Montreal Cognitive Assessment (MoCA)

The MoCA was developed for use in the detection of Mild Cognitive Impairment (MCI), and screens for the common domains of impairment in MCI. The MoCA examines short-term memory recall, delayed recall, visuospatial abilities, executive functions, phonemic and syntactic fluency. Other cognitive functions examined are verbal abstraction, serial subtraction, attention, concentration and working memory and orientation to time and place. These are all examined in a 30-point test which can be administered in approximately 10 minutes. The original MoCA publication sets the cut-off threshold for cognitive impairment as a MoCA score of less than 26. The MoCA has been reported as a valid measure for screening for cognitive impairment and dementia in stroke cohorts, demonstrating higher sensitivity than the Mini Mental State Examination (MMSE), at the cost of lower specificity.

Clinical Neurology Made Easy

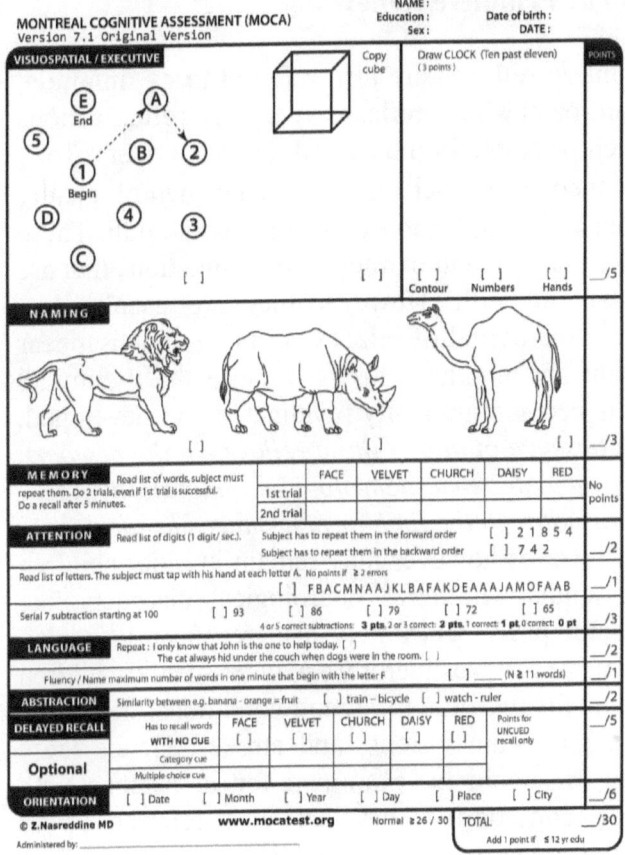

3.5 The Primitive Reflexes

Primitive reflexes are also referred to as infantile, infant or newborn reflexes. They are reflex actions which originate in the central nervous system. They are seen in normal infants, but not neurologically intact adults, in response to particular stimuli. These reflexes are due to extrapyramidal functions that are present at birth. However they are usually lost within the period of infancy. In fact most disappear within six months. This is because the pyramidal tracts become gradually myelinated and developed. *The absence of any of these reflexes in the newborn may indicate some neurological abnormality, local abnormality in the limb or neuromuscular disease.*

The reflexes however may remain in older children and adults who have neurological disorders like cerebral palsy. They may also reappear in adults. Primitive reflexes therefore may be seen in children and adults with the following conditions; dementia, traumatic brain lesions, and strokes. Hence these reflexes should be examined for in persons with these conditions. They are also referred to as frontal release signs. In addition some of these atypical primitive reflexes seem to be an early feature of autistic spectrum disorders.

The common primitive reflexes are as follows;

Asymmetric tonic reflex (Fencing posture)
The asymmetric tonic neck reflex is present at the age of one month. It disappears before the age of six months.

To elicit this, place the child in a supine position and rotate the head to the side, the ipsilateral arm will extend while the contralateral arm will flex (sometimes the motion will be very subtle or slight). There is also a *symmetric tonic neck reflex* which appears and develops around 6–9 months of age and should integrate by around 12 months. Flex the child's head forward, which extends the back of the neck, the upper limbs will flex and the lower limbs will extend. Conversely, when the child's head is extended backward, contracting the back of the neck, the upper limbs will extend and the lower limbs will flex.

Babkin reflex
The Babkin reflex results from different responses to pressure that is applied to both palms. There may be head flexion or rotation, opening of the mouth, or a combination of these responses.

Crossed Adductor reflex
Tap on the quadriceps tendon and note the contraction of contralateral adductor muscles. It is basically a spread of the quadriceps reflex (knee jerk) to the contralateral side. The reflex is present at birth and persists for seven to eight months.

Crossed Extension reflex
The baby should be placed in the supine position. Then one of the legs should pressed firmly down on the bed. Thereafter the same leg which has been pressed down is scratched. The normal response is that the free leg will flex, adduct, and extend. This

reflex is present at birth and disappears after the first month.

Gallant reflex (Truncal Incurvation reflex)
In order to elicit this reflex, scratch the skin of the back from the shoulder downwards. The scratch should be done 2 to 3 cm lateral to the spine. The normal response is a swing of the child towards the side of that is stroked. Hence there is a truncal incurvation. The reflex is present at birth and persists for two to four months.

Glabellar Tap Reflex/Myerson sign
The glabellar is the space between the eyes. The reflex is elicited by tapping the glabellar repeatedly. The normal response is blinking of the eyes. The blinking however stops after two or three taps. In an abnormal (positive reflex) response on the other hand, the blinking continues with repeated taps. This reflex is classically seen in Parkinson disease and may also be seen in other diffuse degenerative diseases like dementia.

Landau (Ventral suspension) reflex
To elicit this reflex, the baby is laid prone on the air. In essence, the baby is suspended in the air. The normal response is that the body the body forms a convex arc upward. In essence, the head, neck, and hips are extended. On the other hand, the shoulders should be drawn back with the legs slightly flexed. This reflex appears at about three months and persists to the age of two years.

Moro reflex (Startle reflex, Embrace reflex)

The Moro reflex is also called the startle reflex because it frightens the baby. To elicit this, hold the baby supine but tilted at 45 degrees. Thereafter allow the head to drop suddenly but gently. The arms will suddenly spread out (abduct, circumduct, as well as extend). The legs will also flex or extend slightly. There is subsequent pulling in of the arms like an embrace (adduction of the arms). In addition, the baby also cries; because of the sudden loss of support. It occurs at birth and disappears between the age of four and six months.

Palmar avoiding response

In eliciting this reflex, the examiner strokes the medial side or dorsum of the hand. The response is a withdrawal of the baby's hand. This may be seen in contralateral parietal lobe disease or its connections.

Palmar Grasp Reflex

Stroke the palm of the hand with a firm object between the thumb and index finger on the radial side. There will be flexion and grasping of the object not inhibited by distracting the patient. Grasping is typically associated with contralateral frontal lobe disease. A similar response occurs on the plantar surface of the foot but it is not as strong.

Palmo-mental Reflex

In the palmo-mental reflex, the stimulation is on the palm while the response is on the chin. To elicit this, quickly scratch the thenar eminence with a key or pin. There is a sudden contraction of the mentalis muscle of the same side of the chin.

Placing reflex
To elicit this response, the baby is held upright while the is put the foot under the edge of a table. Once the dorsum touches the table, the baby will raise the foot and put it on the table. It is usually seen at birth. However, the reflex disappears between the ages of ten months and one year.

Rooting reflex (Search reflex, Point's cardineaux)
Gently rub the infant's cheek; there is exploration of the mother's skin by the newborn mouth in search for the nipple. Therefore, the head turns toward the stimulus, the mouth opens, and sucking begins. The reflex is present at birth and usually disappears by two to three or four months of age. Integrity of the trigeminal system (CN V) is important for the reflex.

Snout Reflex
This is assessed by applying a gentle pressure of the knuckle on the patient's lip. There is reflex puckering of the orbicularis oris.

Stepping (Automatic walk, Dance) reflex
Hold the infant under the arms in a vertical position, once the soles of the feet touches a flat surface they'll attempt to walk by placing one foot in front of the other. This reflex disappears around 5–6 months.

Sucking Reflex
Make a light contact with the cheeks near the corner of the mouth. There will be an anticipatory opening of the mouth as part of released sucking.

Other primitive reflexes are
Finger Extension reflex.
Parachute reflex
Pout Reflex
Swimming reflex

Most of these primitive reflexes cannot be examined in the 60kg adult. The commonest primitive relex that is examined in adults is the glabellar tap reflex. Others are the palmar reflexes, crossed reflexes and the tonic neck reflexes. The sucking reflex may not be examined but you will notice the dementia patient *sucking his food* instead of eating it. In addition, the author has observed that patients with dementia, apart from having the return of these primitive reflexes also tend to lie down in a flexed (fetal) position.

3.6 Asterixis (Liver flap)
Asterixis is derived from Greek (*a* 'not' and *sterixis* 'fixed position'). It used to be called *flappy tremors* because it resembles the flapping wings of a bird.

The name however is a misnomer because it is not a type of tremors. Tremors are classically rhythmic with a two way movement unlike Asterixis which are myoclonic jerks. There is a sudden flexion of the wrists and fingers. To examine, ask the patient to stretch forth the arms and extend the wrist. The patient will be unable to hold the wrist in an extended position which will result in a flap of the wrist. Asterixis is usually seen in metabolic encephalopathies e.g. chronic renal failure, severe congestive heart failure, and acute respiratory failure. Commonly it is seen in decompensated liver failure hence the name (liver flap). It is discussed here because it identifies encephalopathy.

3.7 Conclusion

Examination of the central nervous system starts with a quick general examination usually from the foot of the bed because a lot can be learnt from simple observation. The higher cortical function tests though challenging are examined in details in anybody with features suggestive of a higher cortical dysfunction. However an examination of each cognitive domain is essential for diagnosis. In practice however, most neurologists quickly perform the MMSE.

CHAPTER 4

THE CRANIAL NERVES

4.1 Introduction

There are twelve cranial nerves. All the nerves should be examined systematically. The first and second cranial nerves are actually part of the central nervous tissue rather than peripheral nerves. The third to twelfth nerves arise from the brain stem. They innervate the facial, cranial and cervical tissues. Some of the cranial nerves have motor innervations, some are only sensory and some have both motor and sensory functions.

Remember the pneumonic for the functions subserved by the cranial nerves;

Some (1st) Say(2nd) Marry(3rd) Men(4th) But(5th) My(6th) Brother(7th) Says(8th) Bad(9th) Business(10th) Marry(11th) Money(12th)

S---- The cranial nerve has only sensory supply
M-----The cranial nerve has only motor supply
B----- The cranial nerve has both sensory and motor supply

4.2 Olfactory (First) cranial nerve

In examining the olfactory nerve, the two parameters tested are perception and identification. Commonly used are non-irritant everyday substances like soap, fruits and creams. *Avoid irritant materials because they stimulate the trigeminal fibres in the nasal mucosa.* These materials should be presented to each nostril separately. The second nostril should be closed. The first thing to note is whether the person can perceive smell. The absence of the sense of smell is called anosmia. Local conditions in the nostril like catarrh, sinusitis and nasal disorders are the commonest causes and should be excluded. Some significant causes of anosmia include antibiotics, closed head injury, sub frontal meningoma, meningitic sequalea and HIV Infection. Thereafter, ask whether the patient can identify the particular smell. In parosmia, a pleasant ordour seems offensive. There may be olfactory hallucination in some types of seizures.

4.3 Optic Nerve (Second) Cranial nerve

The optic nerve is one of the most commonly examined cranial nerves. Five parameters are usually tested in the examination of the optic nerve. These are visual acuity, visual fields, colour vision, pupillary reflexes and fundoscopy. Visual localization, visual recognition and motor perception may also be tested.

4.31 Visual Acuity

In the examination of the visual acuity, it is important to ensure that any refractory error is corrected so that ocular disease is recognized. The refractory error however can be overcome by testing reading through a pin which concentrates a thin beam of vision on the macula. Each eye should be tested separately. The visual acuity should be tested before the visual fields.

Distant vision
The Snellen's wall chart is used for distant vision.
The visual acuity is expressed as d/D. D is the distance at which the patient is expected to read the letters while d is the distance at which the patient actually read the letters. A visual acuity of 6/6 is the normal. When vision is better than 6/60, some macular function is present. When the vision is less than 6/60, then the visual acuity is assessed by the patient's ability to count fingers, observe hand movements. If he can neither count fingers nor observe movements, then flash a torch light and see whether he perceives light(light perception). The Snellen chart is not routinely seen in the normal neurology clinic but is seen in the ophthalmology clinic.

Near vision
The Jaeger card labeled J1-J4 is used to test near vision. In the everyday clinic however, the newspaper can also be used for near vision.

4.32 Visual field
The visual field is the whole extent of the sphere of vision in each eye. The visual field is limited by the size of the retina, the margins of the orbit, nose and teeth. It is larger for large objects than that of smaller objects. It is also larger to bright objects than dim objects.The several methods of assessing the visual fields are as follows:

The Confrontation Tests

The confrontation test is the simplest and most practical of all the methods. The patient's field is compared with the examiners field. Both eyes are tested together at first; referred to as binocular. Thereafter, they are tested separately (monocular). This excludes a field defect limited to the field of one eye.

There are two types of confrontation tests: confrontation with a finger and confrontation with the red pin.

Confrontation with a finger

This test maps the whole visual field. Sit opposite (face to face with) the patient at a distance of about one meter. Compare the patient's left eye with your right eye and vice versa. In examining the patient's left eye, ask the patient to close his right eye with his right hand while you close your left eye with your left hand. Thereafter, bring your right index finger or a target in a plane mid way between your faces and ask the patient to follow your finger with his eyes and not the head. It is usually better to stabilize the patient's head with your other hand. Test all the four quadrants separately as you move your finger in an 'H'pattern. Ask the patient to report any diplopia. Thereafter, put your finger at the lateral ends of the patients visual field comparing the patient's visual field is with yours. This examination assumes that your own visual field is normal.

Red Pin Confrontation
The red pin confrontation is a sensitive test for the central field. A 5mm red pin is used instead of the finger. The pin may be mounted on an eraser to remove the examiner's hand out of the field. This method compares the field and the physiological blind spot to the examiner's field. The use of a 2mm pin will define central field defects. Comparing the contour and colour of the palms separately in the fields of each eye could be done for central vision. There will be a difference in the colour intensity in patients with central vision deficits.

Perimetry

The visual field can be mapped quantitatively with the perimeter. These examinations are better carried out by the ophthalmologists in the eye clinic. They are not routinely carried out in the neurology clinic.
 Goldman Perimeter
Tangent (Bjerrum) Screen
Humphrey field Analyzer

Visual Field Abnormalities may present as follows:

Central Scotoma
This is a zone of loss in the center of the field. Unilateral central scotoma is seen in optic neuritis and is feature of multiple sclerosis.
Para central Scotoma
These are caused by disease of the choroid or retina. Vascular lesions commonly cause unilateral para central scotoma. When scotomas are bilateral, they

may be due to toxic causes especially alcoholism and thiamine deficiency. Glaucoma may cause a unique type of para central scotoma.

Hemianopia

This means loss of sight in one visual field. It is homonymous if the same side is involved.

4.33 Colour Vision

The colour vision is tested with the use of pseudo-isochromatic plates with multi-coloured dots. The best known of these plates is the Isihara chart.

The plate is designed in such a way that the patient with an abnormal colour vision will read a different number from the normal patient. The commonest abnormality is the red-green deficiency. The blue-yellow deficiency and total colour blindness are rare. Again, this test for colour vision is usually performed in the eye clinic

4.34 Pupillary Reflexes

There are two types of pupillary reflexes. These are the light reflex and accommodation.

Light Reflex

The light reflex examines both the second and third cranial nerves simultaneously. The light reflex should be examined in a shady indirectly illuminated room. Examine each eye separately. Ask the patient to look into the distance to ensure that accommodation is relaxed and shine a bright light into one eye. Expect the pupil to contract almost immediately, dilate a little again then settle to a smaller size after few oscillations. As you switch off the light, the pupil dilates to its original size. A lesion of the optic nerve will abolish the light reflex on the same side as well as the contralateral eye. Note that there is response in both eyes when you shine light in the normal eye. Also measure the pupil size, shape and observe any asymmetry.

Accommodation/ Near response

To test accommodation reflex, move the target towards the patient's nose. As the eyes converge, the pupils should constrict. *There is usually no need to check this near response (Accomodation) if the pupils respond briskly to light, because an isolated loss of constriction (miosis) to accommodation does not occur.* A commonly used abbreviation to describe normal pupils is *PERRLA* (pupil's equal, round and reactive to light and accommodation). *However, it is important to test the near response if the light response is poor or absent.* Positive response of the pupil to accommodation in the abscence of brisk response to light (*Light-Near dissociation*) however is seen to occur rarely in the following conditions; Argyll Robertson pupil, Parinaud's syndrome and Adie Tonic Pupil (Holmes-Adie Syndrome)

Argyll Robertson pupil

In this condition, the pupils are usually small, irregular, and unequal; fail to react to light and also dilate poorly to my iatric. However, they constrict on accommodation (light-near dissociation). This is known as the Argyll Robertson pupil and is seen in late Neurosyphillis (tabes dorsalis). The condition is rarely seen these days since syphilis has all been eradicated.

Parinaud's syndrome also known as dorsal midbrain syndrome, vertical gaze palsy, or Sunset Sign is an inability to move the eyes up and down. It is caused by compression of the vertical gaze center at the rostral interstitial nucleus of medial longitudinal fasciculus (riMLF).The slightly dilated pupils react on accommodation but not to light (light-near dissociation).

Adie Tonic Pupil (Holmes-Adie Syndrome)
In Adie tonic pupil, the affected pupil is slightly enlarged in ambient light and the reaction to light is absent or greatly reduced. Characteristically, there is light-near dissociation. It may be associated with absence of knee or ankle jerks (*Holmes-Adie syndrome*) and hence be mistaken for tabes dorsalis. Holmes- Adie pupil represents a special form of mild inherited polyneuropathy.

The Swinging flash light test
The *Marcus Gunn pupil* is a relative afferent pupillary defect indicating a decreased pupillary response to light in the affected eye.This is by demonstrated by the swinging flashlight test, where you alternately shine the light into the left and right eyes. A normal response would be equal constriction of both pupils, regardless of which eye the light is directed at. This indicates an intact direct and consensual pupillary light reflex. However in the Marcus Gunn pupil, when you shine the light into the affected eye, there is reduced pupillary constriction

hence the direct pupillary reflex is weaker than the consensual pupillary reflex. This weakness is due to decreased response to light from the afferent defect, while light in the unaffected eye will cause a normal constriction of both pupils (due to an intact efferent path, and an intact consensual pupillary reflex). In essence, the direct and consensual pupillary reflexes are both intact. *This is an important sign in retro bulbar optic neuritis, ischaemic and compressive lesions of the optic nerve.* In some cases, this may be the sole objective evidence for disease. In bilateral optic neuropathy however, *no afferent pupil defect is present if the optic nerves are affected equally.*

Anisocoria

Anisocoria is the presence of inequality in the pupils in response to the light reflex. Subtle inequality in pupil size, up to 0.5 mm, is a fairly common finding in normal persons. In essential or physiologic anisocoria, there is a normal pupillary light reflex. Anisocoria that increases in dim light indicates a sympathetic paresis of the iris dilator muscle.

Anisocoria that increases in bright light suggests a parasympathetic palsy. The first concern is an oculomotor nerve paresis.

The triad of miosis with ipsilateral ptosis and anhidrosis constitutes *Horner's syndrome*, although anhidrosis is an inconstant feature. Horner's syndrome commonly arises from the compression of cervical sympathetic chain by neoplasms, haematoma, abscesses etc. Other causes are brain stem stroke and carotid dissection, but most cases are idiopathic.

4.35 Fundoscopy

The examination of the optic fundus should be carried out in a dark room. The examiner uses his right eye to examine the patient's right eye and vice versa. *You should never go face on with the patient.* Ask the patient to fixate on a far distant object away from the bright light. In routine medical examination in the neurology clinic, it is possible to examine the optic disc and surrounding retina without dilatation of the pupil. In a complete examination of the fundus, the pupils should be dilated by instilling few drops of a mydiatric.

Note that in patients with predisposition to closed-angle glaucoma, an acute attack of glaucoma may be precipitated when the pupils are dilated.

4.4 Occulomotor (Third), Trochlear (Fourth) and Abducens (Sixth)
Ocular Movements

The external ocular movements are controlled by the Oculomotor (third), Trochlear (fourth) and the Abducens (sixth) cranial nerves.

The movements of the eyes include
Abduction; outward movement of the eye (lateral)
Adduction; inward movement of the eye (medial)
Elevation; upward movement
Depression; downward movement
Diagonal; version at any intermediate angle
Rotary; these are not possible voluntarily but are necessary to adjust for mild degrees of head tilt as

in when reading. It could be external rotation which is movement away from the nose or internal which is towards the nose.

The superior and inferior recti act when the eye is in abduction while the superior and inferior obliques act when the eye is in full adduction.

4.41 Inspection

The first thing to note on inspection is the drooping of the eyelids when the eye is completely open (ptosis). Ptosis can be complete or incomplete. The pupil is fixed and dilated when there is third nerve palsy. The response to light in the affected eye is lost but the contralateral eye constricts since its third nerve is still intact. When light is shone into the normal eye, only that normal eye constricts.

4.42 Accommodation

To test accommodation reflex, move the target towards the patient's nose. As the eyes converge, the pupils should constrict.

4.43 Examination of ocular movements

Movements of the eyes are normally symmetrical with the visual axes meeting at the same point. This is called conjugate movements of the eyes. These conjugate ocular movements depend on the brain stem integration of the activity of the nuclei of these three nerves. *Infranuclear lesions of the third, fourth and sixth nerves lead to weakness of individual eye or groups of muscles while supranuclear lesions lead to paralysis of conjugate movements of the eyes.*

To examine the ocular movements, keep the patient's head in a steady position usually by placing your left hand on the head. Then ask the patient to follow an object held at an arm's length. Move the object in your hand at full range of movements both horizontally and vertically. The vertical movements are observed in abduction and adduction. Each eye is examined in six directions. All misalignments and limitations in ranges of movements are noted.

Conjugate movement
The ability of the eyes to move together in the vertical or horizontal direction is referred to as conjugate gaze. Patients with a 3rd or 6th nerve palsy have an obvious squint. These patients usually complain of double vision (diplopia).
Note whether there is a tendency of the gaze to fix in a particular in one particular direction. Upward gaze palsy is also obvious: called sunset eyes.

4.44 Red Glass Test
The red Glass Test is used to assess strabismus. In this rarely performed test, the patient is examined seated. Place a red glass over the right eye and a clear glass over the left. The position at which the patient sees the red image indicates the affected muscle and confirms the squint.

4.45 Nystagmus

The final part is to examine for nystagmus. Ask the patient to look straight ahead and note whether the eye is steady. Patients with albinism have oscillations. Thereafter, let the patient look to the extreme right, to the left, upwards and downwards. It is best to ask the patient to look at the examiner's finger. Examine the rate, amplitude and rhythm of any nystagmus in each direction of gaze. Note the fast phase as well as the gaze when nystagmus is maximal. *Note that physiological nystagmus can occur when the eyes deviate to the endpoint of the gaze.*

4.5 Trigeminal nerve (fifth)

4.51 Examination of the motor function

The Trigeminal nerve has motor functions and also the sensory supply of the face. Observe the wasting and thinning of the temporalis muscle then ask him to clench the teeth. In normal individuals, the temporalis and masseter muscles should stand out with equal prominence on both sides. When there is 5th nerve palsy, the muscles are weak and do not stand out like the opposite side. This is better assessed by palpation. Ask him to open the patient's jaws by applying pressure. When the patient opens his mouth, the jaw will deviate to the weak side been pushed by the healthy lateral pterigoid muscle.

4.52 Sensory Examination

To test the sensory function, pain, temperature, and light touch are examined in the sensory dermatomes of the face. The sensory impairment usually has a

pattern. This could be a root or division pattern or the onion skin pattern. Sensory impairment restricted to one sensory division is in keeping with an extrinsic lesion either from the base of the skull or the deep facial tissues. Intrinsic lesions of the spinal tract of the trigeminal nucleus present the characteristic 'onion skin' appearance. This is because the spinal nucleus is somatotopically organized: its uppermost portion is responsible for perioral sensation, while lower portions serve progressively more peripheral
areas of the face in an "onion-skin" arrangement.

4.53 The Trigeminal Reflexes
The trigeminal nerve also sub serves three reflexes which should be tested. These are:

Corneal reflex
The corneal reflex is the most sensitive indicator of trigeminal nerve damage. Ask the patient to gaze into the distance or ceiling, and then use a wisp of light cotton to touch the lateral edge of the cornea at its conjuctival margin. The patient should blink if the corneal reflex is present. Compare the corneal reflex on both sides. *Note that you should never touch or wipe the cotton with the cotton wisp.* This is because of the danger of ulceration in the presence of corneal anaesthesia. An alternative is to lightly blow a puff of air into each cornea.

Palatal reflex
This is elicited by stimulating the palate. The normal response is swallowing. This swallowing reflex is particularly lost in patients after a Stroke.

Jaw jerk
In order to examine the jaw jerk, ask the patient to relax the jaw. Place a finger on the chin and tap that finger with a hammer. A slight jerk is normal. An increased jerk is seen in bilateral upper motor lesion.

4.6 The Facial (Seventh) nerve
4.61 Examination
The facial nerve is the most commonly examined cranial nerve in my practice because of the high prevalence of stroke in SSA. The first step is to ask the patient to smile or show the upper teeth. The mouth is drawn to the healthy side revealing the presence of facial nerve palsy. There is prominence of the naso-labial folds on the healthy side and absence on the affected side. Thereafter, ask the patient to shut the eyes tightly. The affected eye is not closed at all and if it is, the eye lashes will not be deeply buried. Attempting to open the patients shut eye is almost impossible if the orbicularis oculi is acting normally. A tightly shut eye can only be opened with ease when there is weakness of the orbicularis oculi from facial nerve palsy.

At times, closure of the eye is almost impossible in facial nerve palsy. In such cases, on attempts to forcefully close the eye, the eyeball moves upwards. This is known as Bell's phenomenon. It is actually a normal response but is not seen when the orbicularis oculi is acting normally.

Again, ask the patient to whistle and he will be unable to because whistling is impossible in facial nerve palsy. Another test is to ask the patient to inflate their mouth with air and blow out the cheeks. Air can be made to escape the mouth easily on the affected side by tapping the finger on the inflated cheek.Note the prescence of hyperacuisis in which slight sounds are heard with painful intensity. This exaggeration occurs as a result of the loss of the tympanic membrane damping (an effect of the nerve to the stapedius).

In addition, ask the patient to push out the chin. Palpate the chin and the platysma muscle is will be noted to be weak in facial nerve palsy.

Finally, the sense of taste is tested in the anterior part of the tongue supplied by the chorda tympani .This can be done using sugar or salt. Apply these with a swab or a spatula to the protruded tongue. Ask the patient to indicate whether there is perception of the taste before he withdraws with his tongue. Ensure that the patient rinses the mouth after each test.

4.62 Localizing facial weakness

Lesions of the facial nerve give different types of weakness depending on whether the lesion is above or below the facial nucleus.

Lesions above the facial nucleus cause upper motor neurone or supranuclear palsy while those below cause lower motor neurone or infranuclear palsy. In upper motor neurone lesion, the lower part of the face is chiefly affected hence the patient is able to wrinkle the forehead and shut the eyes tightly. The pneumonic by generations of medical students is *'upper spares upper'*; this means that the upper part of the face is spared. Sometimes only the fibres carrying emotions are affected especially if the lesion is thalamic in origin such that the facial weakness is more evident when the patient smiles. In addition, bilateral upper motor neurone lesions result to emotional lability due to uncontrolled activity of such pathways. Note that taste is not affected and there is no facial muscle atrophy in supranuclear lesions.

In lower motor neurone lesion however both the upper and lower parts of the face are equally affected because the final common pathway is damaged. The taste sensation is lost because the fibres of the chorda tympani are damaged and there may be hyperacuisis because the stapedius muscle is paralysed. There is also associated facial atrophy in lower motor neurone lesions.

4.7 The Vestibulocochlear (eight) Nerve

4.71 Assessment of Hearing

The vestibulocochlear nerve is made up of two components: hearing and balance. Ideally, a crude assessment of hearing impairment can be made during history taking. This is done by asking the patient whether he can hear the door bell or ringing telephone (approx 60 decibels). Ask the patient whether he prefers a raised voice in a quiet environment. The free-field tests are done with practice. The test is done by whispering numbers into one ear (15decibels). Thereafter, the conventional voice is used (50 decibels). If there is hearing impairment, examine the external auditory meatus to exclude wax and infections. Further examination is done by using the tuning fork to differentiate the types of deafness (conductive and sensorineural deafness). A tuning fork with a frequency of 512Hz osr 256 Hz is often used as described below.

Webers Test

In Weber's test, the base of the vibrating fork is placed in the midline like the vertex. The normal response is to hear the sound of the tuning fork more loudly in the midline. This is also the response if hearing is symmetrically reduced. It should not be heard more loudly in one ear. In conductive deafness however, the sound is louder in the affected ear because the distraction from external sounds is reduced. In sensorineural deafness, the sound is louder in the normal ear.

Rinne's test

In Rinne's test, the tuning fork is held against the mastoid process. When the sound disappears, the fork is then held against the external meatus. The patient should hear the sound again since air conduction via the ossicles is better than bone conduction. This is referred to as Rinne positive. This 'Rinne positive' is also the response seen in cases of sensorineural deafness.

In conductive deafness, the converse is true and is referred to as Rinne negative. In essence, the patient does not hear the sound when the fork is held against the auditory meatus (air conduction is not better than bone conduction). Note that patients with small conductive loss may also be Rinne positive. *It is worthy of note that all the clinical tests of hearing have limited reliability hence accurate formal audiometry is essential and carried out in ENT clinics.*

4.72 Assessment of Balance

The examination of vestibular aspect of the eight cranial nerve has a lot of components and is not usually carried out in the clinic. Adequate assessment usually requires specialized investigations. The first step however is to establish whether the vertigo is positional or non-positional. Positional vertigo refers to vertigo that is related to head movements or postures. The presence of positional vertigo usually indicates a canal or nerve injury. Non-positional vertigo on the other hand, suggests an intrinsic brainstem lesion. Other aspects include examination for nystagmus as described above and some specific tests viz Dix- Hallpike test, Unterberger's, Fistula and Rhomberg's tests.

Dix- Hallpike Test

The Dix- Hallpike manoeuvre is important to assess the effect positional change. Ask the patient to sit towards the start end of the examination couch such that his head is outside the couch if he lies down. It is wise to examine the neck movements first to ensure that they are free and painless. Turn the head to 45^0 on the side of the test then rapidly lower the patient to 30^0 below the horizontal. Tell the patient to keep his eyes open and report any sensations of vertigo while you look for nystagmus. Repeat the test in the opposite side. In benign positional paroxysmal vertigo (BPPV), there is a latent period of 5-10 seconds before the onset of vertigo and nystagmus. Note that there is fatigue of this response such that immediate repeat of this shows little abnormality (adaptation). *Persistent positional nystagmus however, implies central pathology.* This is seen in cerebellar, brain stem lesions and disease of the fourth ventricle.

Fistula Test
The fistula test is done when there is evidence of middle ear disease. Here, you compress the tragus into the external meatus. The result is a sense of imbalance and may be accompanied by nystagmus. A positive test implies an abnormal communication between the middle ear and the vestibular labyrinth.

Unterberger's Stepping Test
The patient is asked to stand with outstretched arms. He is then instructed to takes steps on the spot with his eyes closed. There is rotation to the affected side in unilateral vestibular disease.

Rhomberg's test
In Romberg's test ask the patient to stand with the feet together with the eyes open and the hands out stretched. Patients with unilateral labyrinthine disorder will sway to the side of the lesion and this is more marked when the eyes are closed. Meanwhile, those with central lesions sway both sides whether the eyes are open or closed. In posterior column disorders, the patient sways or

even falls when the eyes are closed but doesn't when the eyes are open.

In the gait assessment, ask the patient to walk with the eyes open. You will notice that those with unilateral labyrinthine lesion will veer to one side. The patient with central disorder will stagger a few steps in one direction then veer to the other side.

The Caloric test is rarely performed in recent times. Ask the patient to lie on the couch with head at 30^0 then fix his gaze on a point in the central plane. Irrigate the external canal with water at 30^0 then at 44^0 for 30-40 seconds. Cold water induces nystagmus away from the ear been irrigated while warm water induces nystagmus towards the tested ear *(COWS-cold water opposite, warm water same)*.

4.8 Glossopharyngeal Nerve (Ninth) and Vagus (tenth) nerves

The 9th and 10th cranial nerves are usually assessed together since their actions are seldom individually impaired. These two nerves form the afferent and efferent routes of the Gag reflex (also called Pharyngeal reflex). *Testing the taste sensation in the posterior aspect of the tongue is impractical and is usually not done.*

In the examination, note the patient's voice which may be high pitched in vocal cord paralysis. Note any swallowing difficulty or regurgitation of fluids.

To examine the Gag Reflex, depress the patients tongue with a spatula. The positive response is the elevation of the soft palate and retching (the patient gags). Also ask the patient to say 'ah' while depressing the tongue with a spatula and note any asymmetry of palatal movements.

4.9 Accessory (Eleventh) Nerve

In assessing the accessory nerve, ask the patient to rotate the head against resistance because the sternocleidomastoid turns the head to the right and vice versa. Compare the power and muscle bulk. Thereafter ask the patient to shrug the shoulders and hold them in this position against resistance. The patient should be able to manage any attempt to depress the shoulders. Also compare the power and muscle bulk on both sides.

4.11 Hypoglossal (Twelfth) Nerve

In examining the hypoglossal nerve, ask the patient to open his mouth and inspect the tongue. Tremors of the tongue are noted in Parkinson disease whether the tongue is protruded or at rest. Is there evidence of atrophy? This is noted by increased folds and wasting of the tongue. Are there fasciculations? Wasting and fasciculations are features of lower motor neurone lesions. *Bilateral fasciculation is almost pathognomonic for motor neurone disease.*

Thereafter, ask the patient to put out the tongue as far as possible.

In unilateral hypoglossal lesion, the tongue is been pushed to the weak side instead of been protruded straight. Note that a deviation of the mouth caused by facial nerve paralysis may occur. To differentiate, ask patient to move tongue from side to side to lick the cheek. Note whether this can be done freely.

4.10 Conclusion

Examination of the cranial nerves is an important aspect of the nervous system examination. It also requires a logical order just like parts of the nervous system examination. The more you examine all the cranial nerves, the easier it becomes. In practice, the commonly examined cranial nerves are the 2nd, 3rd, 4th, 6th and 7th nerves. Proper examination localizes the lesion to either the brain or the peripheral nervous system.

CHAPTER 5

MOTOR SYSTEM EXAMINATION

5.1 Introduction

The motor system (which provides the motor functions of the body) is probably the most popular part of the nervous system being the most obvious. The impairments of motor function may be subdivided into (1) paralysis due to an interruption of lower motor neurons, (2) paralysis due to dysfunction of upper motor (cortico-spinal) neurons, (3) apraxia or non-paralytic disturbances of purposive movement due to involvement of association pathways in the cerebrum, (4) involuntary movements and abnormalities of posture due to disease of the basal ganglia, and (5) abnormalities of coordination (ataxia) due to lesions in the cerebellum. Hence the motor system should be examined having these components in mind. In practice however, lesions of the cortico-spinal tracts (pyramidal tracts) usually to take preeminence because of the impairment of power.

5.2 Appearance
Examination should always start from the foot of the bed. The first thing to look out for the presence of any asymmetry of movements, attitude of the limb or deformity in the limbs. This is especially important in persons who are unable to communicate or unconscious. Such a person may be moving only one side of the body (scratching,

cleaning his face, gesticulations etc) irrespective of the side that is stimulated.

This asymmetry indicates that there is weakness of the other side. Note that in infants, the preference of one hand which is referred to as handedness is developed at the 1 year. *Consequently, a child under one year will always bring out the two hands simultaeneously on an attempt to receive a toy. Bringing out one hand for an infant is considered a type of asymmetric movement.* It means that there is a problem with the other arm which may be from the bone, joint or nervous system. It could also be just a bruise, a boil or cellulitis and not necessarily weakness. Also take note of the attitude of the limbs. The normal limbs should be in the anatomical position when a person is lying supine. This means that the heels down with the toes pointing up. A weak lower limb on the other hand will be laterally rotated with the toes pointing side wards. Deformity of the limb or limbs suggest fractures.

5.21 Bulk of muscles

The bulk of muscle is best assessed by inspection and palpation. Carefully inspect the muscles and note whether there is muscle wasting or hypertrophy. When in doubt, measure the circumference at a fixed distance above or below the point. Note the pattern of muscles involved in the wasting. Is the wasting generalized? Generalized muscle atrophy may not likely to be caused by neurological disorders. It is seen in cachexia of any cause (Malnutrition, Malignancies,

HIV/AIDS, Tuberculosis, Protein loosing enteropathies, Thyrotoxicosis etc). Wasting of muscles is also a normal feature of aging. Are the muscles involved upper or lower limb muscles. Is it wasting symmetrical or asymmetrical. Which muscle groups are involved: proximal muscles, distal muscles, small muscles of the fingers?

Does the wasting involve a particular nerve root like in weakness of the extensor muscles of the ankle (foot drop)? Muscular atrophies involve specific muscle groups (shoulder and pelvic girdle muscles). Thereafter, palpate the muscles. Atrophied muscles are usually smaller, soft and flabby when they are contracted. When accompanied by fibrosis, they are hard and inelastic. Hypertrophied muscles are bigger and firmer to touch. True hypertrophy occurs in response to continued excessive workloads like in athletes and certain occupations like the military from years of training.

Furthermore, examine for fasciculation which is an irregular, non rhythmical contraction of muscle fascicles. It increases with exercise and can be elicited on tapping the muscle surface. Muscle myokymia is a rapid rippling of muscle fibres. This is particularly in the orbicularis oculi but occasionally in large muscles. It occurs after exercise or with fatigue. Also note whether there are abnormal movements like tremors, dystonias, chorea and myoclonic jerks.

5.3 Tone of muscles
The tone refers to resistance to passive movement across the joint. It is a state of tension or contraction

found in healthy muscles. An increase in tone is called hypertonia and a decrease is hypotonia. This is examined by moving the limbs passively across various joint. The maintenance of tone is dependent on the spinal reflex. Assess the tone by moving the joint through its range of movements. The elbow is a hinge joint so flex and extend the joint to check whether the tone is normal, decreased or increased.

The wrist has a wide range of movements: flexion/extension, pronation/supination and circumduction so move the joint through the whole range. In examining the tone across the hip which is a ball and socket joint, place both hands on each thigh and roll it from side to side (roll the ball in the socket). The knee is another hinge joint and should be examined accordingly. The ankle like the wrist also has a wide range of movements: plantar flexion/dorsi flexion, inversion/ eversion and circumduction. Once again, move the joint through the whole range. Note that during the examination you should also compare the right side with the left. Physiologic hypotonia is seen in sleep. Some pathologic causes of hypotonia are lower motor neurone lesions, sensory neuropathies, cerebellar disease and some medications (hypnotics, antispasmodics).

Common causes of hypertonia (rigidity) include pyramidal lesions (like Stroke), dystonias, Parkinson disease, Dementia and muscles across a painful joint.

There are three types of rigidity: clasp knife, lead pipe and cogwheel rigidity. Clasp knife and lead pipe are elicited with the flexion and extension movements. In clasp knife rigidity, flexion is free but extension is rigid. This is classically seen pyramidal lesions (like Stroke). In lead pipe rigidity, both flexion and extension are rigid. Cog wheel rigidity is only elicited at the circumduction movements of the wrists and ankles. It feels like a chain going over the teeth of the wheel; occurs because of the combination of rigidity and tremors in the limb. Lead pipe and cogwheel rigidity are features of Parkinson disease.

5.4 Power/ Strength

The assessment of power is easily done by watching the patient walking, standing, standing up from a sitting or lying position. Also watch the patient is while dressing or undressing and jumping lightly or hopping. Ask the patient to perform all these movements while he is on bare foot. Observe all these movements carefully as they will test the proximal and distal strength as well as coordination.

5.41 Pronator/Parietal Drift

Pronator drift is performed when a pyramidal (UMN) weakness while being suspected is not obvious as the patient is observed as described above. Ask the patient to hold the hands outstretched with the hands in supination for up to one minute. Ensure that the eyes closes his eyes in order to prevent visual compensation. You will notice that the weaker arm pronates and gradually drifts downwards. This test detects subtle pyramidal weakness.

The Medical Research Council grading of power

Grade 0   Complete paralysis
Grade 1   A flicker of contraction only
Grade 2   Ability to move with gravity eliminated
Grade 3   Movement against gravity
Grade 4   Movement against resistance
Grade 5   Normal power

This scale is clinically based, easy to reproduce, but non linear. It requires practice in order to be reproducible.

Grades 1, 2 and 3 assess small differences in very quick muscles. Grade 4 contains a wide variation in strength. Grade 5 is normal but subjective and varies between age groups, gender, physical development and the health of the patient. Expectedly, the young are stronger than the elderly, men are stronger than women and the healthy are stronger than the ill.

5.52 Examination of Gross power

Traditionally, start the examination for gross power by asking the patient to lift the limb. If the patient is able to lift the limb, this means that the power is at least grade 3 (able to move against gravity). Thereafter, assess grades 4 by placing your hand to resist the patient's already raised limb to see whether he can lift it further against your resistance. Ability to lift the limb to some extent against your resistance is considered grade 4 power while the power at its fullest is considered grade 5 power. *Note that differentiating between grades 4 and 5 is mainly subjective.* When the patient can lift the limb against resistance; most neurologists will note that 'power is at least 4'.

However, on asking the patient to lift the limb, if he is unable to lift the limb, this means that the power is less than 3 (unable to move against gravity). Therefore, go ahead and assess grade 2 by asking the patient to move the limb from side to side (horizontal movement). If he is able to move the limb horizontally the power is 2. If he is still not able to move the limb horizontally, ask the patient to flick the fingers. If he is able to flick the fingers or toes, that is grade 1 (flicker of movement).

If there is no flicker movement, the power is zero. Grade 1 -4 is referred to as *paresis* while grade 0 power is referred to as *plegia*.

Mono refers to one limb while *hemi* refers to involvement of both the upper and lower limbs on the same side. *Quadri* or *tetra* refers to the involvement of all four limbs while *tri* refers to three limbs. Involvement of two symmetrical limbs if referred to as *di (para* for the two lower limbs and *brachial di* for the two upper limbs*)*. Hence hemiplegia means grade 0 power on one side while hemiparesis means between grades 1-4 power on one side. Paraplegia means grade zero power in the two lower limbs while paraparesis refers to grades 1-4 power in the lower limbs. Other deficits are named accordingly.

5.5 Testing Of Individual Groups

There may be need to test the individual groups especially in peripheral neuropathies. When testing these individual groups, think of nerve root and supply. The individual groups are examined as follows:

5.51 Upper Limbs
Shoulder
Stabilization of the scapula (C5, 6, 7)
This is the function of serratus anterior. Ask the patient to push the wall. If there is paralysis, the scapula is winged.

Trapezius
The upper part is tested by asking the patient to shrug the shoulders while the examiner tries to press down from behind.

For the lower part, the patient tries to approximate the shoulder blades.

Shoulder abduction (C 5, 6)
This function is carried out by the deltoid and the supraspinatus. Ask the patient to abduct arm against resistance.

Shoulder adduction (C 6, 7, 8)
This is the function of the pectoralis major, latismus dorsi and the teres major. Ask the patient to bring the arm to the horizontal. Hold the elbow and resist shoulder adduction.

5.52 Elbow
Elbow flexion (C5, 6)
This is the function of the biceps. Ask the patient to flex an arm in full supination against resistance.

Elbow extension (C, 7, 8)
This is the action of the triceps. The patient is asked to straighten out the forearm against resistance.

5.53 Forearm

Forearm supination (C6, 7)
Grasp the patient in a hand shake with the elbow extended and resist supination.

Forearm pronation (C6, 7)
Also grasp the patient in a hand shake with the elbow extended but resist pronation.

Brachioradialis (C5, 6)
Ask the patient to flex arm against resistance in mid position between pronation and supination.

5.54 Wrist and hand

Finger extension (C 7, 8)
Ask the patient to extend fingers against resistance.

Thumb extension (C 7, 8)
Ask the patient to extend the thumb against resistance.

Finger flexion (C 7, 8)

Try to extend the patient's flexed terminal phalanges. You can also ask the patient to squeeze your index and middle fingers.

Thumb opposition (C 8, T1)
Ask the patient to touch the base of the 5th finger with the thumb against resistance.

Finger abduction (C8, T1)
Ask the patient to abduct each finger against resistance.

Wrist extensors
Weakness of the extensor muscles leads to wrist drop. Ask the patient to make a fist. Attempt to forcibly flex the wrist against the patient's effort to maintain the posture.

Wrist flexors
When there is weakness of the wrist and the fingers the person is unable to make a fist. Ask the patient to make a fist around your first two fingers. Ideally, you should be unable to withdraw your fingers from a normal hand-grip. If you are able to withdraw your fingers, the hand grip is weak.

5.54 Neck flexors
Ideally, a person should flex the neck freely such that his chin should touch his chest. *Flexion of the neck is a particularly sensitive marker for proximal myopathy.* The patient is unable to flex the neck against your resistance if the neck flexors are weak.

5.55 Muscles of the trunk

The paralysis of the abdominal muscles is detected by the displacement of the umbilicus when the patient attempts to rise. When there is paralysis of the lower segment, the umbilicus moves upwards. This is referred to as 'Beevor's sign'. If the upper segment is affected, the umbilicus moves downwards. When there is severe weakness of the abdomen and hip flexors, the patient is unable to rise without the aid of the hands. If the hands are not used, the legs lift up 'Barbinski rising up sign'. This does not occur in hysterical patients who are able to rise with ease ('Hoovers' sign).

5.56 The Diaphragm

A simple test is to ask the patient to take a deep breath and then count slowly. Most people can count up to 20 or more with a single breath. A patient with diaphragmatic paralysis will not be able to count up to 20.

There is also difficulty in taking a brief sniff. This is because the sniff requires maximal diaphragmatic contraction.

Spinal extensors

Extension of the spine is the function of the erector spinae and muscles of the back. The patient is asked to lie prone. You will note that the neck and back are extended. The muscles of the back stand out if they are healthy.

5.56 Hip

Hip adduction (L 2, 3, 4)
The patient lies on the back with the hips abducted. Ask the patient to push the knees together against resistance.

Hip abduction (L 4, 5, S1)
The patient lies on his back with the legs placed together. Ask the patient to abduct the thighs against resistance.

Hip flexors (L 1, 2, 3)
Ensure that the thigh is flexed to a right angle and then ask the patient to flex further against resistance. Another way is to extend the patient's leg on the bed then ask him to raise the leg off the bed against resistance.

Hip extensors (L 5, S1, S2)
The patient's knee is extended and is lifted off the bed. Thereafter ask him to keep the heel on the bed against resistance. This is normally a very strong movement and should be impossible to overcome in a normal patient.

A better functional test is to observe the patient standing from a low chair and hopping.

5.57 Knee
Knee extensors (L2, 3, 4)
Flex the patient's knee. Hold the knee and ask him to extend it against resistance.

Knee flexors (L5, S1, and S2)
The patient lies supine and the knee is flexed at right angle. Hold the leg at the ankle and resist pulling of the leg towards the buttock.

5.58 Ankle and foot
Plantar flexors/Ankle extensors (S1, 2)
This is the function of the gastrocnemius. The patient lies supine with the legs extended. Ask the patient to plantar flex against resistance.

Dorsi flexors/Ankle flexors (L 4, 5)
This is the function of the tibialis anterior. The patient lies supine with the legs extended. Hold the foot and resist dorsi flexion.

Ankle inversion (L4, 5)
This function is sub served by the tibialis posterior. Hold the patient's foot medially at the first metatarsal and resist inversion.

Ankle eversion (L5, S1)
Hold the patient's foot laterally and resist eversion.

Toe extension (L 5, S1)
The patient dorsi flexes the toes against resistance.

Toe flexion (L5, S 1, 2)
The patient plantar flexes the toes against resistance.

5.58 Patterns of Limb weakness and possible diagnostic submission;

	Location of Weakness	Features	Diagnosis
1	Proximal and Axial Weakness	Weakness of the shoulder and pelvic girdle muscles	Primary Muscle Disease
2	Pyramidal (Unilateral or bilateral)	Weakness of the leg flexors more than the extensors, Weakness of abduction of the arm	Pyramidal lesion like stroke, brain malignancy or other focal CNS lesions
3	Distal location	Weakness of the small muscles of the hands and feet	Polyneuropathy
4	Focal	Weakness in the distribution of a single nerve or nerve root	Mononeuropathy or plexopathy
5	Global	Generalized weakness and wasting	Systemic disease e.g. Chronic diseases like TB, HIV, Malnutrition Malignancy, ETC
6	Random	Weakness at multiple sites	Mononeuritis Multiplex, May be an evolving systemic disease.

5.6 Deep Tendon Reflexes

A tap on the tendon with the patellar hammer (tendon hammer) causes a sudden stretch of the muscle. This is called the deep tendon reflex. The loss or reduction of this reflex suggests a sensory nerve or root lesion. Exagerated deep tendon reflex is significant if it is asymmetric or if there are other signs of upper motor neurone lesions. Other common causes are Thyrotoxicosis and Tetanus. Increased or brisk reflexes however are not always pathologic and may be seen in anxiety states.

The following are important skills in eliciting the reflexes;

Patient should lie at ease with the genitalia covered.

Patient should be warm and comfortable.

The technique should be standardized e g, using the same patellar hammer.

Reassure the patient.

Repeat the test if necessary.

Occassionally, the tendon reflexes can only be elicited by reinforcement which increases anterior horn cell excitement. Hence, when the reflex is lost absent, ask the patient to make a strong voluntary muscular effort. This may be interlocking the fingers together while attempting to pull apart, clenching the teeth or making a strong fist then tap the tendon again with the patellar hammer. This reinforcement is called the *Jendrassik* manoeuvre. If there is no response after this reinforcement, then the reflex is indeed lost. Diminished or absent tendon reflexes are seen in peripheral nerve disorders, Poliomyelitis, Hypokalaemia, trisomy 21 and acute stroke.

Deep tendon reflexes are graded as follows
Grade 0   Absent
Grade 1   Present (as in a normal ankle jerk)

Grade 2   Brisk (as in normal knee jerk)
Grade 3   Very brisk
Grade 4   Clonus

5.61 Method of examination
Jaw jerk (5th nerve)
Ask the patient to relax the jaw. Place a finger is placed on the chin and tap with the patellar hammer. A slight jerk is normal. An increased jerk is seen in bilateral upper motor lesion.

Biceps jerk (C5, 6)
Place the patient's arm in a relaxed and flexed position across the trunk. Leave the forearm is in semi prone position. Palpate the biceps tendon with your index finger and strike it firmly with the hammer.
The biceps will contract.

Supinator jerk/Brachioradialis jerk (C5, 6, 7)
Place the elbow in a slightly flexed and slightly pronated position. Strike the hammer on the styloid process of the radius. This will cause supination of the forearm, with flexion of the elbow and fingers.

Inverse Supinator jerk
This occurs in patients with mid cervical lesions (C5, 6). The full supinator jerk as described above is not seen instead, the biceps jerk (C5, 6) will be absent. The supination and flexion components of the Supinator jerk will also be absent. Brisk flexion of the fingers (C7) occurs instead. *The author thinks*

that the more appropriate name should be incomplete Supinator jerk.

Triceps jerk (C6, 7, 8)
Slightly flex the arm. Strike the hammer on the triceps tendon above the olecranon process after palpating the tendon. The triceps will contract. *Do not strike the belly of the muscle.*

Hoffman's reflex (C7, 8)
The Hoffman's reflex is also called the *finger flexion reflex*. Flick or tap the nail of the terminal phalanx patient's third or fourth finger. The flexion of the terminal phalanx of the thumb constitutes a positive response and indicates a cortico-spinal tract lesion. The Hoffman reflex was once called the upper limb Barbinski reflex.

Knee jerk (L2, 3, 4)
The knee jerk is the first tendon reflex to become part of regular neurological examination. The patellar hammer derives its name from this reflex. The patient lies supine. The knees are relaxed and flexed to less than 90^0. Pass your hand under the knees (above the popliteal fossae) to support ensuring that the two knees do not touch. Strike the hammer mid way between the origin and insertion of the patellar tendon. Observe the contraction of the quadriceps. This can also be done with the patient sitting at the edge of the bed and the legs hanging freely.

Ankle jerk (S1, 2)

Externally rotate the patient's leg. This places the foot at 90^0 to the calf and the calf at 90^0 to the thigh. Slightly dorsi flex the ankle to stretch the Achilles tendon. Strike the tendon on the posterior surface. Watch for calf contraction and plantar flexion. This can also be elicited when the patient is kneeling on the chair with the Achilles tendon above. *Ankle jerk is lost early in Diabetic neuropathy.*

5.62 Ankle Clonus

The ankle clonus is an indication of hyper reactivity of the ankle stretch reflex. Note that in the grading of reflexes above, clonus is the highest grade of exaggerated reflex. In essence, the deep tendon reflexes must be increased before clonus can be elicited. Clonus therefore confirms markedly increased deep tendon reflexes. In testing for clonus, ensure that the patient is relaxed in the supine position. Slightly flex the knee with your palm above the popliteal fossa and then suddenly dorsi flex the foot.

There is production of a series of oscillatory beats at the rate of about 3/s. A few (<3) of these oscillations could be normal. When they persist (more than 3), it is referred to as *sustained clonus*. It is seen in upper motor neurone lesions. A similar response can also be seen in the patella and elbow (patella and elbow clonus respectively).

5.7 The superficial reflexes

The superficial reflexes are polysynaptic reflexes which are elicited in response to cutaneous stimuli. They do not depend on muscle stretch receptors. The abdominal and plantar reflexes are particularly important.

5.71 Corneal and Palatal reflexes (5th nerve)

These two reflexes arise from the fifth cranial nerve.

The corneal reflex is the most sensitive indicator of trigeminal nerve damage. Ask the patient to gaze into the distance or ceiling, and then use a wisp of light cotton to touch the lateral edge of the cornea at its conjuctival margin. The patient should blink if the corneal reflex is present. Compare the corneal reflex on both sides. *Note that you should never touch or wipe the cotton with the cotton wisp.*

This is because of the danger of ulceration in the presence of corneal anaesthesia. An alternative is to lightly blow a puff of air into each cornea.

The palatal reflex is elicited by stimulating the palate. The normal response is swallowing. The swallowing reflex is particularly lost in patients after a Stroke

5.72 Scapular reflex (C5-T1)

The scapular reflex is elicited by stroking the skin between the scapular. The scapular muscles will contract.

5.73 Superficial abdominal reflex (T7-12)
The patient lies supine with the abdomen exposed. Drag a thin wooden stick quickly and lightly across the abdomen. Ensure that this is done dermatome by dermatome from the loin towards the midline. You will notice a ripple of contraction of the underlying musculature. These are absent in upper motor neurone lesions. *These abdominal reflexes are difficult to locate in obese or multi-parous women.* They are brisk in anxious patients.

5.74 Cremasteric reflex (L1, 2)
The cremasteric reflex is carried out in men. Stroke the skin at the upper inner part of the thigh. The normal response is that the testicles move upwards.

5.75 The plantar reflex (L5, S1)
The plantar response is the most commonly examined of all the superficial reflexes probably because of ease of access to the plantar surface. In addition to this, it is also an objective response that can be compared by various observers. The plantar response is important in identifying upper motor neurone lesions. Place the patient in a supine position and ensure that the muscles of the lower limb are relaxed. Thereafter, stimulate the outer edge of the sole of the foot firmly by scratching a key or stick along it from the heel towards the little toe. Most doctors use the tip of the patellar hammer for the stimulation. The normal response should be the flexor response which is plantar- flexion of the big toe.

An abnormal response is made up of extension (dorsi-flexion) of the big toe preceding all other movements. This is referred to as the extensor plantar response. In more severe cases, this response is followed by extension and fanning out of all the other toes, marked dorsi-flexion of the ankles and finally flexion withdrawal of the hip and knee. The constellation of the extensor plantar response, fanning out of all the other toes and withdrawal of the limb is referred to as the 'Barbinski response'. *Note that in infants less than 1 year, extensor plantar response is the normal response.* The flexor response appears in the subsequent 6-12 months as myelination of the corticospinal tracts is completed. Bilateral extensor response is pathognomonic for upper motor neurone lesions.

There are other methods of eliciting the plantar response as follows:

Allen-Cleckley sign
Apply a sharp upward flick and sudden release of the second toe. Pressure over the ball of that toe may also be applied.

Bing sign
Prick the dorsum of foot with a pin; could be done multiple times

Chaddock reflex (lateral malleolar sign)
Scratch the skin below the lateral malleolus from behind forward. The reversed Chaddock sign is

elicited by scratching the skin from the front backward.

Cornell sign
This is elicited by scratching the inner side of the dorsum of foot or extensor hallucis longus.

Gonda-Allen sign
Flex then suddenly release the distal phalanx of the second or fourth toe downwards.

Gordon sign
Squeeze the calf muscles.

Moniz sign
This is elicited by passive plantar flexion of the ankle.

Oppenheim reflex
A heavy pressure is applied with thumb and index finger to the anterior surface of the tibia, over the shin, from knee to ankle.

Schaffer sign
Pinch the Achilles tendon.

Stransky sign
Pull the little toe laterally and suddenly release it.

Strümpell sign
Apply a forceful pressure by the finger and thumb down the anterior tibial spine.

Thomas reflex
This is elicited by rubbing the sole of the foot with the back of the knuckles two or three times.

Throckmorton sign
Tap over the dorsum of the first meta-tarso-phalangeal joint just medial to the extensor hallucis longus tendon.

The comparative yield of twelve methods used to elicit the extensor plantar reflex shows that the classic method, Gonda-Allen, Allen –Cleckley, Chaddock and Cornell methods gave the highest values.

5.8 THE GAIT

The gait is the manner in which a human can move, either naturally or as a result of specialized training. The gait is best examined when the patient is not aware so that he does not make adjustments as you observe him walking. In a clinic setting, it is wiser to examine the gait while the patient is walking into the clinic. The following gaits are the identified abnormal gaits.

Apraxic/Frontal lobe gait
The apraxic gait is seen in frontal lobe disease. The patient walks slowly and the step length is greatly shortened. The base is also slightly wide because the patient is protective. There is difficulty in initiation of movement (appears glued to the ground) and also in stopping the movement.

The power is normal because there is no weakness of the muscles. The pathology originates from the motor association cortex.

Atasia-Abasia/Hysterical gait
This gait is bizarre with no pattern. Hence, it can take any form and has no defined pattern. Characteristically, the patient walks normally when the examiner looks away. The patient has a tendency of falling into the examiners arms. Further examination will reveal neither motor nor sensory abnormalities. This unusual gait is seen in women with hysteria.

Cerebellar Ataxic /Drunken Sailor Gait
The cerebellar gait also called the drunken sailor gait is a broad based gait. Characteristically, the patient's feet are wide apart. He is unable to put his feet together and is unsteady. There is also an erratic shifting of weight from one side to the other. In essence, the person walks like a drunken man. This is seen in patients with cerebellar dysfunction hence the name. Further examination will reveal impaired tandem walk.

Dystonic gait
The patient with dystonia is slow with a distorted posture (One of the author's patients with axial dystonia walked into the clinic looking backwards). The step length is normal and the base is erratic. There are twisting athetoid movements which interrupt walking. This is classically seen in axial dystonias and particularly in dystonia musculorum.

Festinant/Parkinsonian gait
The patient may initially be slow until festination sets in. It is characterized by *short rapid shuffling* steps; because the steps are quickened, he leans forwards as he tries to catch up with the centre of gravity. There is associated reduced or total absence of the arm swing. The patient is slow on turning (En-bloc movement). This is classically seen in Parkinson disease.

Foot drop/Slapping gait
In this gait, the cadence, step length and base are normal. There is however an over lifting and slapping of the foot because the ankle flexors are very weak. The ankle joint therefore seems excessively loose and the toes get to the ground first (slap the ground). The heels barely touch the ground. In isolation, this gait indicates a common peroneal nerve injury or an L5 lesion with foot drop. It is also seen in Charcot-Marie Tooth disease.

Gladiator gait
There is marked stiffness and rigidity. The step length is short. The name is derived from the gladiators seen in Roman films. This gait is seen in patients recovering from tetanus who are generally very stiff. It is also seen in Stiffman's syndrome.

Hemiplegic gait

The hemiplegic gait is seen in patients with pyramidal lesions. On the affected side, the arm is flexed across the chest with the leg extended. There is circumduction and scraping of that affected leg. This is the commonest gait abnormality in the author's environment giving the fact that stroke is very common in the African Negro and many survivors have this gait abnormality.

High Steppage/ Stamping
The patient is also unsteady like the cerebellar gait hence ataxic. It is also slightly broad based with short step length. The patient seems to be unaware of the distance to the ground and hence uses excessive force resulting in stamping. This gait is seen classically in patients with distal symmetric poly neuropathy (DSPN).

Marche a' petit Pas/Aging
There is an alteration of gait unrelated to overt cerebral disease that accompanies aging. The main characteristics are a stooped posture, varying degrees of slowness, stiffness of movements and shortening of stride. There is no arm swing. They walk with caution and lean slightly forwards.

Myopathic /Waddling gait
The waddling gait is seen in patients with proximal myopathy involving the pelvic girdle especially the gluteal and hip abductors (weight bearing muscles). These weight bearing muscles are no longer able to support the pelvis against the pull of gravity. The rhythm and step length are normal and the base is

broad. There is over lifting of the hips making the patient waddle like a duck. This gait is best observed from behind.

Para paretic/Scissors gait

The patient walks on a narrow base with the knees, slightly flexed (like a pair of scissors). There is plantar flexion such that the toes scrape the floor with associated circumduction of the hip while the stepping leg is being lifted forward. The gait is classically seen in spinal cord disease or bilateral pyramidal lesions and also in children with cerebral palsy. Some authors refer to this gait as the spastic gait.

Toppling gait

In this gait, there is tottering and falling. This occurs in brain stem and cerebellar lesion especially in elderly patients who had a stroke. It is frequent feature of lateral medullary syndrome in which the patient falls to the side of the infarction. It may also occur in patients with vestibular neuronitis where the patient falls to the side of the lesion.

Trendelenburg gait

The patient walks with a limp and leans heavily to one side. There is also over lifting of the hip. It is some sort of unilateral waddling. This gait abnormality is seen in patients with *unilateral* hip injury or weakness of hip muscles as in poliomyelitis and also commonly seen in tuberculosis of one hip.

Vestibular gait
This may be seen in patients with acute uncompensated vestibular lesion. The patient is noted to lurch to one side while moving.

Cautious Gait
Cautiousness is seen in the elderly as noted above. However, it is very common when vision is impaired. Hence it is classically seen in the blind and also when there is darkness.

5.9 Conclusion
The examination of the motor system is the most popular aspect of the nervous system examination. This is because of the impairment of power is worrisome to patient since their everyday activities are remarkably impaired. The deficits are also easier to appreciate. Examination of the gait is extremely revealing and is one of the easiest ways to make a diagnosis.

CHAPTER 6

THE SENSORY EXAMINATION

6.1 Introduction
A sensory modality is an experience recognized by the individual as unique. The special senses are vision, taste, hearing and smell. Most of the special sense have been discussed above as part of cranial nerve examination. The other superficial senses perceived on the skin are tested by the bedside.
These are
Pain
Temperature
Vibration
Joint position sense
Tactile sensibility
Stereognosis

Sensory perception depends on the physiological interaction of afferent inputs at different levels in the nervous system. Sensation is broadly classified into epicritic and nociceptive.

Epicritic are those enter the nervous system through the large myelinated fibres. The nociceptive on the other hand, enter the nervous system through thinly myelinated or unmyelinated fibres. For clinical purposes, vibration and joint position sense belong to the epicritic group while pain and temperature belong to the nociceptive group. Light touch belongs to both groups and as such is not helpful in distinguishing large versus small fibre disease. Light touch is also not helpful to differentiate diseases of the posterior column and that of the spinothalamic tract. the impairment of light touch connotes a global involvement.

6.2 Examination

Most neurologists consider examination of sensation the most difficult part of neurological examination. This is partly because of the required patient's cooperation. Moreover, the examiner must also be aware of the sensory dermatomes and peripheral nerve distribution of the whole body. This knowledge is necessary to appreciate that a certain distribution of abnormal sensation results from a lesion of a particular peripheral nerve, nerve root or spinal segment. Often times, no objective sensory loss can be detected despite symptoms of sensory disturbance. This is because sensory symptoms in terms of parasthesias and dysesthesias may be due to axons which are not sufficiently diseased to cause deficits. *Rarely, the opposite may occur where deficits are noted in patients with no sensory symptoms.*

6.3 The sensory dermatomes

There are pictures of the sensory dermatomes but they are best remembered as follows:

Brief summary of the Sensory Dermatomes

	Face	Trigeminal nerve
	Vertex	Trigeminal nerve
	Occiput	C2
	Neck	C3

	Deltoid/Shoulders	C4
	Biceps and upper lateral forearm	C5
	Lower lateral forearm and 1st two fingers	C6
	Middle finger	C7
	Last two fingers	C8
	Upper Medial forearm	T1
	Medial Biceps	T2
	Male Nipple	T4
	Xiphisternum	T6
	Umblicus	T10
	Symphisis Pubis	T12
	Groin	L1
	Thigh	L2
	Knee and surroundings	L3
	Shin, medial leg and medial malleolus	L4
	Lateral aspect of the leg and 1st four toes	L5
	Small toe, plantar and posterior leg	S1
	Posterior thigh	S2
	Saddle area	S3, S4 and S5

The saddle area consists of concentric rings around the anus when sitting astride like on a saddled horse hence the name (saddle area). The outermost ring is S3. The next ring is S4 while the innermost ring is S5.

6.4 Testing of sensory modalities
6.41 Pain

A simple method of testing this important modality is by using a sterile pin prick. Use a pin that is sharp enough to cause a painful pricking sensation rather than pressure. Usually, a hat pin is used, but then hats that need pins are no more in vogue and are not easily accessible. Ordinary office pins can be used as a substitute. *Note that hypodermic needles are never used since they are designed to pierce the skin.*

Delineate the areas of abnormality by moving from the area of reduced sensation to a normal zone and not the other way round. *A distal loss is more common than a proximal loss. It is therefore wiser to start distally and progress proximally hence sensory examination is about the only part of the examination where you examine from down –up.*

The first thing is to demonstrate on a likely normal area like the forehead or the back of the neck to establish the expected sensation. Start at the side of the tip of the digit and gradually move up: dermatome by dermatome with the limb in anatomical position. The patient should have his eyes open since pain cannot be seen because closing his eyes may make him anxious or sleepy. The patient therefore may lose concentration and give spurious answers. Keeping the eyes open will not affect the result except in the joint position sense. Avoid repeating the test more than once since repetition causes fatigue. The skins of the palmar and plantar surfaces are usually thickened especially in patients that do a lot of manual labour and are therefore not tested because they are insensitive.

In patients with suspected distal symmetrical polyneuropathy (DSPN), having examined the pain modality dermatome by dermatome as described above, start again from the tip of the digit and inch proximally while asking the patient where the sensation changes. This is generally referred to as 'inching'. This should be carried out in both the hands and feet. This may delineate the 'glove and stocking' pattern seen in distal symmetric neuropathy. This is classically seen in Diabetic neuropathy.

6.42 Pressure
This may be tested by squeezing the Achilles' tendon (*Abadie's* sign). This was popular when tertiary syphilis was common especially in tabes dorsalis. It is still used in patients in deep coma. There are other sites for eliciting pressure. These include compressing the ulnar nerve against the ulnar bone (*Pitre's* sign), applying pressure on the eyeballs (*Haneal's* sign) and squeezing the testis (*Biernacki's* sign).

6.43 Temperature
Testing the temperature sense seldom provides additional information because pain and temperature run in the same tracts and provide similar. If required however, it can be tested by using test tubes or beakers containing warm and cold water. The part of the body to be examined is touched and the patient says whether it feels hot or cold. More commonly, at the bedside, temperature is examined with a tuning fork or the end of an ophthalmoscope (cold metals) which gives a rough assessment. Temperature sense is also examined dermatome by dermatome from down–up.

6.44 Tactile Sensibility/ Light touch

Light touch is usually examined with a wisp of cotton wool. The stimulus is first applied to the normal part of the body to acquaint the patient with the nature of the stimulus. Ask the patient to say yes when he feels the stimulus. He is also asked whether it feels different from the normal site. The touch may be reduced or increased.

It may also be perceived as painful, burning, tingling or irritating. Deft application of the examiners finger tip (usually the index finger) or even the patient's own finger tip has been suggested by some authors. Areas of diminished or abnormal sensations should be delineated and recorded. This is also done dermatome by dermatome from down-up. In patients with suspected distal symmetrical polyneuropathy, having done the above, you also start from the tip of the digit and inch proximally to delineate the 'glove and stocking' pattern as described in pain examination.

More precise testing is possible by using a von Frey hair. In this method, a stimulus of constant strength can be applied. Thereafter, the threshold for tactile sensation is determined. This is done by measuring the force required to bend a piece of hair of known length. There are limits in testing the tactile perception. This happens when a series of stimuli cause a decremental response. This is either through adaptation of the end organ or because the initial sensation outlasts the stimulus and also seems to spread. In this situation, the patient may fail to report tactile stimuli in an area where it was present.

He may also report the contact without being touched.

6.45 Vibration sense

Vibration sense is tested with a tuning fork with a frequency of 128 Hz, because vibrations of a higher frequency are more difficult to perceive. Place the foot of the vibrating fork on a bony prominence. This could be the dorsum of the large toe, the medial maleolus, and tibia, dorsum of the finger or the tip of the shoulder.

Note that these bony prominences also correspond to the sensory dermatomes. The patient indicates when he feels the vibration and as it fades in intensity until it ceases. If the examiner can still feel it, then the vibration sense is impaired. If there is impairment, the examiner moves proximally. Vibration sense is a semi-quantitative test and is of value in early demyelinating diseases. It is also impaired in peripheral neuropathies and posterior column disorders. *Vvibration sense is the first sensory modality to be lost in DSPN from Diabetic neuropathy.*

6.46 Proprioceptive sense

Awareness of position and movement of the limbs, fingers, toes are the two modalities that comprises proprioception. These two modalities are usually lost together. There are some clinical conditions however where the position sense is lost but movement is retained. *The perception of passive movements is first tested in the fingers and toes because, when the defect is present, it is reflected maximally in these parts.* The important thing is to grasp the digit firmly by the sides at 90° to the plane of movement because if not, the pressure you apply may allow the patient to note the direction of movement. This also applies to testing the more proximal aspects of the limb. Instruct the patient to report each movement as being 'up' or 'down' from the previous position. This is known as directional kinesia. Thereafter, he is asked to close the eyes, look away or shield the eyes wither bed sheet while the digits are moved while he responds.

Note that this is the only part of sensory examination where the patient is asked to close or shield his eyes. Move the part being tested rapidly. It is important not to move the digits in a rhythm (up-down, up-down) because the patient will get used to the rhythm and you will get a false positive result. The sensitivity of the testing is enhanced by using the third and fourth fingers and toes. Normally, a very slight degree of movement is appreciated in the digits. This can be as little as one degree of an arc. Repeat the test enough times to eliminate chance which is seen in as much as 50% of responses. The defective perception of passive movement is judged by a normal limb if unilateral. In the cases of a bilateral defect, this is judged by the examiners observation. Rapid movements are more easily detected than the slower ones. Inattentiveness causes some of the errors observed.

6.5 Cortical sensation
When these sensory functions are normal and a cortical lesion is suspected, further examination is carried out. These are
Two-point discrimination
Sensory inattention
Stereognosis
Graphaesthesia

6.51 Two point discrimination
The ability to discriminate between two points is a useful quantitative measurement. Use a pair of blunt dividers, apply them simultaneously and painlessly. Then ask the patient whether he feels one point or two different points.

The distance at which the stimuli can be recognized as a distinct pair (two different points) varies.
It is roughly:
1 mm at the tip of the tongue
2-3 mm on the lips
3-5 mm at the finger tips
8-15mm on the palm
20-30mm (2-3cm) on the dorsum of the feet
4-7cm on the body surface

The two point discrimination is an excellent objective sensory test and is particularly useful in patients with lesions of the sensory cortex who may mistake two points for one. It is also useful in posterior column lesions. In some peripheral nerve lesions, like the carpal tunnel syndrome, large afferent fibres are involved and impair discriminatory sensation.

6.52 Sensory inattention

Sensory inattention is an important feature of lesions of the parietal lobe. Ask the patient is asked to close his eyes having explained the procedure so that he does not get anxious. Stimulate or touch simultaneously homologous points on opposite sides of the body with a pin prick. Thereafter ask the patient to indicate which side or sides you touched. The stimulus on the abnormal side is not perceived in sensory inattention. This is also called sensory extinction or neglect. *Note that sensory inattention can be confused with hemianaesthesia.*

In order to differentiate both, some neurologists have suggested moving the limb from the affected side to the normal side which improves the recognition of the stimulus in sensory inattention with no improvement in hemianaesthesia.

This movement however is not always feasible because of pain or spasticity. Another suggestion is to ask the patient to voluntarily familiarize themselves with the abnormal side and then reapply the stimulus and see whether there is improved recognition. The author uses other methods, like asking the patient to draw the face of the clock and see whether he will only draw half the face or the history of eating the food on one side of the plate, colliding with the door or objects on the affected side; these are in keeping with sensory inattention.

6.53 Stereognosis

Stereognosis connotes the ability to identify an object by palpation. Objects commonly used are marble, paper clip, keys or coins. Ask the patient to differentiate different objects without looking. The objects should be felt with one hand at a time. Individuals who are unable to identify common objects placed in their hands have astereognosis.

6.54 Graphaesthesia
Graphaesthesia is the recognition of numbers or letters traced on the skin. These letters should be larger than 4 cm on the palm and should be drawn with a sharp pencil. On the pulp of the finger, numbers as small as 1 cm can be detected. Inability to recognize these numbers is called agraphthaesia. Note that graphesthesia, stereognosis, and extinction cannot reliably be tested for unless primary sensation is intact bilaterally. Hence there should be a full examination of the primary sensory modalities before assessing for cortical sensory loss.

6.6 Conclusion
The sensory examination is challenging because the full cooperation of the patient is required. Care should be taken in explaining the examination to the patient. A good knowledge of the sensory dermatomes is cardinal in the interpretation of the result.

CHAPTER 7
OTHER EXAMINATIONS

7.1 Introduction

There are other examinations that are specific to certain disease in the central nervous system. These are specific examinations carried out to localize the lesions. The cerebellum is part of the motor system but has specific tests to ascertain its involvement.

7.2 Meningeal Irritation

7.21 Neck stiffness

The neck can be noted to be stiff from wrong postures. Neck stiffness however is defined as the resistance to the flexion of the neck. *Resistance to neck extension or side-ways movement is not considered neck stiffness.* Ask the patient to flex the neck as fully as possible to ascertain the degree of movement possible and thereafter relax. Ideally, the chin should touch the chest without pain in normal persons. You can also passively flex the neck especially in the unconscious patient. In meningeal irritation, neck flexion causes pain in the posterior part of the neck which may radiate to the back. Neck stiffness is almost pathognomonic for meningitis but is also seen in subarachnoid haemorrhage, cervical spine disease and in lesions in the posterior fossa and foramen magnum. In extreme cases of neck stiffness, there may be neck retraction though this is rare; it was formerly a feature of untreated tuberculous meningitis particularly in children.

The retraction could be so severe the child is severely bent backwards and looks like a tripod (tripod sign); in which case the retracted neck feels like a third limb. Neck stiffness is very sensitive in unconscious patients; having more reliability that Kernig's sign.

7.22 Kernig's sign

The Kernig's sign is elicited while the patient is in the supine position. Flex the thigh on the abdomen while the knee is already flexed; thereafter attempt to extend the knee. This attempt to passively extend the knee elicits pain and spasms of the hamstrings. The spasm of the hamstring muscle should be demonstrated by palpation.

7.23 Brudzinski's sign

The Brudzinski's sign is also elicited while the person is lying supine. Here, a passive flexion of the neck will lead to a spontaneous flexion of the hips and knees. In fact, it is wise to look out for the Brudzinski sign while examining for neck stiffness. Kernig's and Brudzinski's signs are not very sensitive especially in unconscious patients. They may also be absent or reduced in the extremes of life, in immune-compromised patients and in those with severely depressed mental status. *Neck stiffness is more sensitive.*

7.3 Tests of Coordination/ Cerebellar function

Smooth motor activity requires the coordination of different muscles or groups of muscles. If coordination is impaired, motor performance becomes difficult or even impossible. This impairment is referred to as ataxia. It is important to watch the patient dressing or undressing, handling a book or picking pins. In essence these complex but regular everyday movements are often very sensitive in the assessment of coordination.

7.31 UPPER LIMBS

Finger nose test
The finger nose test is important is the assessment of dysmetria(difficulty with lengths / distances). In the examination, the patient is asked to touch the point of his nose with the index finger. Thereafter, he should touch a target (usually a pen or spatula) that is held up at a distance. He does these movements (to and fro) repeatedly. The test should be carried out on both sides. Normally, the to and fro movement should be smooth. There should be no and the person should be able to touch the target. In patients with cerebellar disease, there is difficulty. This may be in the form of overshooting the mark also called hypermetria or past pointing. There could also be undershooting the mark also called hypometria. In addition, the movements are irregular.

The examiner can also ask the patient to drop an object on the table. The person may bang the object because on the table having made a wrong estimation of the distance to the tabletop. In some cases, the limb may actually stop midway. In addition and the target can only be met with jerky movements. In fact, the author noted a particular patient who could not clap. Both hands were arrested and jerked forwards and backwards as they could not meet the target (the other hand). You can also ask the patient to use his hand to trace a square or draw a circle in the air. The circle will be smooth and circular in a normal persons. In a patient with cerebellar dysfunction, the circle is irregular.

Dysdiadochokinesis
Testing for dysdiadochokinesia is another useful test in cerebellar ataxia. Ask the patient to make rapidly alternating movements like pronation and supination of the forearm. In dysdiadochokinesia, the movements are slow, awkward, irregular and incomplete. In fact, it is often impossible after a few attempts. These rapid movements can also be tested in the fingers by asking the patient to rapidly touch each finger in turn with the thumb and index fingers. Once again, note the awkwardness, irregularity and incompleteness of the movements.

7.32 LOWER LIMBS
Heel shin test
The heel shin test is the lower limb version of the finger-nose test. Ask the patient to lie supine on the bed. Thereafter, the person should put one heel on the shin of the other knee and run it down the shin till it gets to the ankle. Once again, the patient

should carry out this to and fro movement repeatedly. The test should be carried out on both sides for comparison. These movements should be smooth. In cerebellar disease however, the movements are irregular and slow. In addition, instead of a slide down the sheen, the heel swings from one side to another. The test should be performed with the eyes open. You can also ask the patient to draw a large circle in the air with the big toe.

Walking
Observe the patient as he walks into your clinic. You will notice that the patient will deviate off the straight line. There is associated unsteadiness as the patient turns to walk back. The patient may have the classical cerebellar ataxic gait as described earlier.

Finally, ask the patient to 'tandem walk'. In tandem walk, the person is asked to walk on a straight line. One foot is placed in front of the other without space in between the feet. the person walks as though he or she is walking on a tight rope. You will notice that he is unable to being awkward, irregular and may actually fall to one side.

OTHERS
Rhomberg's sign
The Rhomberg's sign is actually a test for loss of position sense not cerebellar dysfunction. Ask patient to stand with feet close together and then close his eyes. You will notice that the patient is

able to maintain his balance when his eyes are open; however, he sways as soon as the eyes are closed and may even fall. The essential feature of the sign is that there is unsteadiness while standing with the eyes closed. On the other hand, there is no unsteadiness when the eyes are open. The test is positive in posterior column lesions or tabes dorsalis. It is more difficult in labyrinthine and cerebellar disorders.

7.4 The Autonomic Nervous System
The autonomic nervous system is a part of the nervous system that controls the normal activities of muscles of the heart, the intestinal tract as well as the glands.

Examination of the autonomic nervous system

7.41 Pupillary Reflexes
The pupillary reflexes are the normal reflexes of the eyes. The first is the Light reflex. The light reflex should be examined in a shady indirectly illuminated room. Each eye should be examined separately. Ask the patient to look into the distance to ensure that accommodation is relaxed. Thereafter, shine a bright light into one of the eyes. The normal response is the contraction of the pupil almost immediately. Then the pupil dilates a little again before it settles to a smaller size after few oscillations. On switching off the light, the pupil dilates back to its original size. Note that there is response in both eyes when you shine light in the normal eye. Also measure the pupil size, shape and

observe any asymmetry. *There is usually no need to check the near response if the pupils respond briskly to light, because an isolated loss of constriction (miosis) to accommodation does not occur.* A commonly used abbreviation to describe normal pupils is *PERRLA* (pupil's equal, round and reactive to light and accommodation).

There are certain pupillary abnormalities observed. These abnormalities may be transient or permanent and may therefore, be discovered only with repeated observation.

Some persons with autonomic dysfunction may have alternating anisocoria

Adie's pupil is larger than normal and responds poorly to light and slowly and incompletely to accommodation. This abnormality results from interruption of parasympathetic innervation of the eye.

Certain pharmacologic agents could be instilled into the conjunctiva. These medications could help to determine the locus of autonomic abnormality in a patient with miotic pupils or abnormal pupillary responses to light. Instilling 1% solution of hydroxyamphetamine or 4% solution of cocaine into the conjunctiva will cause dilatation of the pupil. Neither agent will dilate the miotic pupil if the locus of autonomic dysfunction is postganglionic.

7.42 Sweating Abnormalities

Take time to inspect the skin. The casual observation of sweating patterns during the course of an examination may suggest autonomic abnormalities. Note whether there is total absence of sweating (anhidrosis) in an extremely warm environment, absence of sweating in isolated areas, or the restriction of profuse sweating to the upper body while sweating in the lower body areas is absent. Also note whether there is profuse sweating associated with the ingestion of food (gustatory sweating). Such sweating abnormalities have been commonly associated with the autonomic neuropathy of diabetes mellitus.

Horner's syndrome, consisting of a constricted pupil (miosis), droop of the lid (ptosis), and lack of or diminished sweating (anhidrosis), is occasionally observed in autonomic dysfunction. While inspecting the skin, also note the presence of tropic changes like absence of hair growth.

7.43 Cardiovascular Reflexes

The pulse rate generally increases in the following conditions: exercise, fear and in anxiety states. The pulse decreases at rest and during sleep.

In autonomic dysfunction however, there is tachycardia at rest and the usual slowing of pulse with deep inspiration and in response to Valsalva manoeuvre is absent.

There is also abscence of the normal increase in blood pressure on standing and in performing stressful tasks like mental arithmetic. The absent response of the blood pressure on standing may be severe enough to cause orthostatic hypotension.

Orthostatic/ Postural Hypotension

An important evaluation of normal autonomic control of the cardiovascular system is response of the blood pressure and pulse rate to changes in posture. Ask the patient to lie supine for at least 2 minutes before recording the blood pressure and pulse rate. Thereafter let the patient stand erect for 8-10 minutes and measure the blood pressure again. Ensure that you carefully observe the patient during this exercise in order to prevent hypotension to the point of syncope. You need aassistance to hold the sphymanometer at the level of the heart and also prevent injury to the patient if he falls. Should syncope occur, the patient must immediately be placed in the head down, legs elevated position to restore cerebral perfusion? Also note the heart rate because the failure of heart rate to increase with the development of symptomatic orthostatic hypotension is indicative of autonomic dysfunction.

7.5 Spine

7.51 Inspection

On inspection of the spine note the presence of redness, a wound or fracture. Look for any gibbus which is s feature of vertebral collapse classically seen in Potts disease. Are there any discolourations or tufts of hair which may be a feature of spins bifida in children? In ankylosing spondylosis, the whole spine is stiff and the person is unable to sit down. Slightly box the vertebral column to elicit any tenderness indicative of a possible fracture.

The normal thoraco-lumbar spine is S-shaped. Note the presence of any curvature. The curvature could be anterior, posterior or lateral. Anterior curvature is called lordosis and is normal in the cervical and lumbar areas. Posterior curvature is referred to as kyphosis: slight normal kyphosis in the thoracic spine. This normal should be distinguished from the pathological gibbus which may be caused by Pot's disease, fractures or malignant deposit on the spine.

The lateral curvature of the spine which may be towards either side is referred to as scoliosis.

7.52 Movements of the spine

Cervical Spine

The movements of the cervical spine are tested as follows;

Rotation; Ask the patient to look over the shoulders one at a time.

Flexion; Ask the patient to touch his chest with his chin.

Extension; Ask the patient to look up to the ceiling.

Lateral Bending; ask the patient to bend the neck to the side and attempt to touch the shoulder without lifting the shoulder.

During these movements, note whether there is pain or parasthesiae especially with sustained extension or lateral flexion. Such features are in keeping with nerve root involvement. Examine for wasting and weakness of the muscles thereafter.

Thoracic and Lumbar spine

The main movement of the thoracic spine is rotation while that of the lumbar are flexion and extension. Examine the thoracic and lumbar spines as follows:

Flexion: Ask the patient to touch the toes without bending the back.
Extension: Ask the patient to bend backwards.
Lateral Bending: Ask the patient to run the hand on the side of the thigh to as far as possible.

Thoracic rotation: Ask the patient to sit with his arms crossed. Thereafter, he should twist to the left and then to the right as far as possible. *It is worthy of note that a rigid lumbar spine should always investigated for a serious pathology viz infection (Staphylococcal or Tuberculosis), malignancy or inflammation like Ankylosing spondylitis.* Spinal movements are virtually absent in ankylosing spondylitis.

7.6 Tests for Myasthenia Gravis

There are bedside tests carried out in persons with suspected myasthenia gravis (MG). They help to make a diagnosis of MG in resource poor settings like in SSA where the Tensilon is not easily available and affordable.

7.61 Counting test

Ask the patient to take a deep breath then count up to 50. The voice should be normal with the same loudness and timbre. However, in a person with myasthenia gravis, the voice reduces gradually as he counts till he becomes inaudible. This is as a result of the fatiguability.

7.62 Curtain test
In the curtain test, ask the patient to sustain an upward gaze. A normal individual should be able to sustain an upward gaze for about one minute, in MG however, the patient is unable to sustain an upward gaze for 15 seconds. The upper lids just fall like the horizontal venetian blinds hence the name (curtain test).

7.63 Ice pack test
The ice pack test is commonly carried out in patients with bilateral ptosis. *Note that bilateral ptosis is considered to be caused by Myasthenia Gravis until proven otherwise*. Ask the patient to lie down. Place ice cubes in cellophane packs over his closed eyes. Allow the packs to stay for five minutes before removing them.

You will notice that thereafter, the eyes which were drooping suddenly open well and the patient will also be able sustain an upward gaze.

7.64 The Snarl test
Ask the patient to smile. The smile is classically a snarl because of the weakness of the muscles of facial expression.

7.65 The Sleep test
The sleep test is taking from the history of marked improvement after sleep. You can also ask the patient who is very weak to lie down and sleep for

30 -60 minutes. There is remarkable improvement in the muscle strength when he wakes up.

7.66 Arm abduction test
Ask the patient to abduct the arms and sustain in the horizontal position for one minute. You will notice that the patient with MG is unable to sustain the arm in abduction for 10-15 seconds.

Any of these tests; counting, curtain, snarl, arm abduction test can be repeated after the Tensilon test. There will be remarkable improvement of strength in these prior weak muscles after the injection of Tensilon; in essence, the person will be notably able to count, sustain an upward gaze, smile without a snarl and sustain arm abduction.

7.7 Entrapment Neuropathies

7.71 Tinel's sign
Tinel's sign is also called distal tingling on percussion. It is a test that examines compressed nerves. Lightly tap over the nerve with a patellar hammer. This will elicit a sensation of tingling or "pins and needles" in the distribution of the nerve. In Carpal Tunnel Syndrome at the point where the median nerve is compressed at the wrist, Tinel's sign is often "positive" causing tingling in the thumb, index, middle finger and the radial half of the fourth digit. It can also be positive in tarsal tunnel syndrome. It is also positive in the compression of the ulnar nerve at the wrist (Guyon's canal syndrome). In this case, the tingling

is felt on the ulnar half of the fourth digit and the fifth digit.

7.72 Phalen's manoeuver
Phalen's manoeuver is another test for detecting carpal tunnel syndrome. Ask the patient to hold his wrist in complete and forced flexion. Thereafter, push the push the dorsal surfaces of both hands together for 30–60 seconds. This will cause the characteristic symptoms such as burning, tingling or numb sensation over the thumb, index, middle and ring fingers. The test however is not very sensitive.

7.73 Oschner's clasp test /Pointing test
Ask the patient to clasp the hand together while the fingers are interlocking. In this case, due to the weakness of flexor digitorum profundus, the index finger will fail to flex and rather point hence the name (Pointing test). It is also positive in Carpal Tunnel Syndrome.

7.74 Tourniquet's test
Tie a sphygmomanometer which is pumped above the systolic pressure for 2 minutes. Once again there may produce the symptoms (tingling) on the affected arm in median nerve palsy.

Lhermitte's Sign (Barber chair phenomenon)

Lhermitte's sign is also referred to as the Barber chair sin. This signifies the bending of the head while sitting on a chair in the barber's during a haircut. Hence the patient is asked to bend the head forward. Another method is to pound on the posterior cervical spine while the neck is flexed. The patient will feel an electric sensation down the back and into the arms. The sign usually indicates that there is a compression of the upper cervical spinal cord or lower brainstem. Some of the conditions that cause a positive Lhermitte's sign include multiple sclerosis, transverse myelitis, Behçet's disease, trauma, radiation myelopathy, vitamin B12 deficiency (subacute combined degeneration). Others include the compression of the spinal cord in the neck from any cause such as cervical spondylosis, disc herniation, tumor, and Arnold-Chiari malformation.

Conclusion

These examinations are specific for specific conditions but then are not carried out routinely by many doctors despite being important parts of the neurological examination. These however can be very enlightening depending on the history. Features of meningeal irritation are probably the most popular of these series of examination. The tests of cerebellar dysfunction are also easy to carry out by the bedside and in routine neurology clinics.

CHAPTER 8

EXAMINATION OF THE UNCONSCIOUS PATIENT

8.1 Introduction

Examination of the unconscious patient is considered difficult by most doctors. This is mostly because there is lack of patient cooperation in these patients. Moreover, the history in an unconscious patient may be unreliable as noted in the chapter on history taking. The unreliable history and lack of cooperation make the examination more challenging but not impossible. The key to proper examination is once again a logical order.

8.2 General Examination

The general examination of the unconscious patient is very important and therefore should not be limited as it may reveal important diagnostic signs. The following are quickly noted

8.21 Appearance

The patient's general appearance is very revealing. Is the patient clean, well nourished and catered for or unkempt? A patient who is clean and well dressed, adorned with jewelries, make-up and perfume usually indicates an acute lesion like acute ischaemic stroke or brain haemorrhage of any cause. Check whether the person is wearing a bracelet.

Persons with certain disorders like Epilepsy, Diabetes Mellitus, and Addison's disease usually wear a bracelet indicating their diagnosis. This will narrow down the possible differentials of the unconsciousness. Is he dirty, disheveled or malnourished? A dirty appearance (as though he rolled on the floor), bruises on the face and buccal cavity and urine smell are in keeping with seizures. Chronic alcoholics, intravenous drug users, homeless and indigent persons will be disheveled and malnourished. Check for needles points which may indicate that the patient is an intravenous drug user or on regular injections like Insulin or Heparin giving an indication of the previous diagnosis.

8.22 Temperature
Check the patient's temperature. Fever suggests a systemic infection, bacterial meningitis or encephalitis. On rare occasions, it may indicate a brain lesion with disturbance of the temperature regulating centers like sub-arachnoid or intracerebral haemorrhage. Hyperpyrexia is seen in cases of heat stroke, anticholinergic drug intoxication and neuroleptic malignant syndrome. Hypothermia may be observed with alcoholic, barbiturate, sedative or phenothiazine intoxication. It may also be seen in hypoglycaemia, severe sepsis, cardiac arrest, hypothyroidism and circulatory failure.

8.23 Respiration
Quickly note the respiratory rate as tachypnoea may indicate acidosis or pneumonia. Abnormal patterns

of respiration may be noted in the unconscious patient. These include Cheyne-Stoke respiration, Kussmaul respiration and apneustic respiration.

8.24 Pallor

Quickly check if the patient is pale? Pallor may be a feature of an earlier diagnosis like a malignancy or chronic kidney disease especially if the patient also has edema. Pallor should be assessed repeatedly. *Increasing pallor indicates internal haemorrhage or sequestration.*

8.25 Ordours

There are certain characteristic ordours that may be perceived. Noteworthy is the uraemic fetor (ammonia/urineferous smell) seen in uraemic patients, the fetor hepaticus (fishy smell) in hepatic encephalopathy. Others are the acidotic breath diabetic ketoacidosis and other causes of metabolic acidosis and finally the Almond smell of cyanide poisoning. Also note whether there is a smell of alcohol. Persons after an epileptic fit may also have a urine or fecal stench if the patient had urine or fecal incontinence during the epileptic fit.

8.26 Evidence of bleeding

The patient may have petechial haemorrhages and ecchymoses. These suggest thrombotic thrombocytopenic purpura, meningococcemia or viral haemorrhagic fever. Ebola virus disease was an epidemic in West Africa few years ago and Lassa fever is actually endemic in Nigeria. Echymoses may also arise from a bleeding diathesis, disseminated intravascular coagulation with subsequent intra cerebral haemorrhage.

8.27 Evidence of trauma

Check whether there is evidence of trauma? Bruising or laceration of the scalp may be seen. Facial and buccal wounds (mainly biting of the tongue) are particularly characteristic of seizures. There may be scalp edema or haematoma which can be palpated. Bruising of the scalp behind the pinna called *'battle sign'* is an important sign of middle fossa or temporal skull fracture. Periorbital haemorrhage which is called *'raccoon eyes'* and bleeding from the external auditory meatus are also reliable signs of basal skull fracture. Fractured limbs are usually noted in abnormal positions.

8.28 Others

Note the prescence of jaundice, liver palms and stigmata of chronic liver disease which are in keeping with hepatic encephalopathy. There may be rashes seen in meningococcaemia. Edema may be a feature of cardiac, hepatic or renal disease.

Are there needle marks on the arms? These are seen in · intravenous drug users or persons on sub cutaneous medications. Are there any septic spots?

8.3 Cardiovascular Examination

8.31 Pulse and blood pressure

These are not part of the usual general examination. They are however of utmost importance in the unconscious patient and may be the difference between life and death hence their inclusion here.

An increase in the pulse rate is seen in hypovolaemic shock from bleeding, fluid loss or any other cause. It could also be a feature of an infectious process like meningitis or sepsis. Other causes include pulmonary infarction, acute myocardial infarction, cardiac tamponade and in fact cardiogenic shock.

Pulse is usually thready, and in some cases totally absent. The pulse rate may be low in raised intracranial pressure and myxoedemal coma.
Marked hypertension indicates hypertensive encephalopathy or a rapid rise in intracranial pressure. It may also occur acutely after a head injury.
Hypotension is characteristic of coma from internal haemorrhage, myocardial infarction and severe sepsis. Hypothermia is also a feature seen in alcohol, barbiturate intoxication, and adrenal crises and in syncopal attacks.

8.4 Nervous System Examination

8.41 Observation
The first thing to do is to observe the patient from the foot of the bed. Patients who toss about, reach up towards the face, cross their legs, yawn, swallow, scratch, cough or moan are close to being awake. The lack of movement on one side of a limb which is usually laterally rotated suggests hemiplegia; there is asymmetric limb movement of the normal side. Intermittent twitching movements of a finger, toe or facial muscle may be the only

sign of seizures (subtle seizures). *Multifocal myoclonic jerks are almost always due to a metabolic cause.* The commonest metabolic cause from this author's experience is Hyperglycaemic Hyporosmolar state. Myoclonic jerks are also common in uraemia, anoxia or drug intoxication.
Haloperidol and lithium are particularly notorious. Rarely, myoclonic jerks are also noted in HIV/AIDS. Hashimoto disease and spongiform encephalopathy are very rare causes. For a patient who is drowsy, bilateral asterixis which is a form of myoclonus is a feature of metabolic encephalopathy or drug intoxication.

8.42 Posture
The posture of the patient is often revealing. These postures may occur spontaneously or be elicited by sensory stimulation. In decorticate rigidity or posturing, there is flexion of the elbows and wrists with supination of the arm. This suggests bilateral damage rostral to the mid brain. In decerebrate posturing there is extension of the elbows and wrists with pronation. This indicates damage to the motor tracts in the midbrain or caudal diencephalon. Less frequently, there may be a combination of arm extension with leg flexion or flaccid legs. This combination is associated with lesions in the pons. These concepts are adapted from animal work and are not very précis in humans. In practice, acute and widespread cerebral disorders, regardless of the location, frequently cause limb extension. In due time, almost all extensor posturing eventually become flexor.

8.43 Level of Arousal and Elicited Movements

Assess the level of arousal. The conversational volume of voice is used. If there is no response, other increasing stimuli are used. Other ways are calling the patient's name, loud noise and sudden flashes of light. The nostrils could be tickled with a wisp of cotton. This is a moderate stimulus to arousal.

All patients except deeply comatose patients will move the head away and rouse to some degree. If the patient uses the hand to remove the offending stimulus, the degree of responsiveness is greater.

Noxious stimuli could be applied or deep pressure.

8.44 Consciousness

Once again, consciousness is assessed with the Glasgow coma as follows:

Table : Glasgow Coma Scale

Eye Opening	Verbal Response	Motor Response
Spontaneous 4	Oriented 5	Obeys Command 6
To Call 3	Confused 4	Localizes Pain 5
To Pain 2	Inappropriate 3	Withdraws to pain 4
None 1	Incomprehensible 2	Abnormal Flexion 3
	None 1	Abnormal Extension 2
		None 1

Once again, the best score is 15 and the lowest is 3 representing none in all the categories. Patients with a score of 8 have good prognosis.

During examination, the motor response may vary. Abnormal extension implies decerebrate posturing. Supraorbital pain may produce extension response while finger nail pain produces flexion. One arm may localize pain while the other may flex. When this occurs, the better response is recorded. This correlates better with final outcome. Asymmetric limb response may be noted in a patient with hemiparesis. Some writers suggest only the use of the arm response for conscious level assessment. This is because leg response to pain is less consistent. Note that movements may be produced from the spinal origin than the cerebral cortex.

The GCS however has a few draw backs.
Patients with aphasia and quadriplegia are scored lower than their real score. This is because the aphasia is mistaken for poor verbal response. In the same vein, quadriplegia is also mistaken for poor motor response. Patients with a tracheotomy tube who are unable to speak are scored as number T (8T or 6T). Some of the patients may have their eyes open and staring into space. For these patients, the eye is threatened and if the patient blinks, he is scored 4. If he doesn't, then the score is 1. The blink is a brainstem reflex.

8.45 Brainstem reflexes

Assessment of these reflexes is essential to localization of the lesion in coma. *Coma is usually ascribed to a bilateral hemispheric disease when brain stem reflexes are preserved.* The converse however is not always true i.e. abscence of the brain stem reflexes does not necessarily connote the abscence of bilateral hemispheric lesion.

The brain stem reflexes conveniently examined are
Pupillary light responses
Spontaneous and elicited eye movements
Corneal responses
Respiratory pattern

Pupillary response

These are the light reflex and accommodation. The light reflex is easily examined in an unconscious patient. Accommodation is not examined however since it requires the patient's cooperation.

Light Reflex
The light reflex examines both the second and third cranial nerves simultaneously. It is done in a shady indirectly illuminated room. Each eye should be examined separately. A bright light is shone into one eye. The pupil is expected to contract almost immediately, dilate a little again then settle to a smaller size after few oscillations. When the light is switched off, the pupil dilates to its original size. A lesion of the optic nerve will abolish the light reflex on the same side as well as the contralateral eye. When light is shone in the normal eye, there is response in both eyes.

Normally reactive pupils essentially exclude midbrain damage. Reaction to light is often difficult to appreciate in pupils 2mm in diameter. If the pupils are unequal (*anisocoria*), a decision as to which is abnormal must be made. About 12% of normal individuals have physiological inequality. Such physiologically unequal pupils react normally to light. An unreactive and enlarged pupil (6mm) or one that is poorly reactive signifies a compression or stretching of the third nerve of a mass above. Occasionally, the smaller pupil may be to *Horner's* syndrome. An oval and slightly eccentric pupil is a transitional sign that accompanies early midbrain-third nerve compression. Bilaterally dilated and unreactive pupils represent the most extreme pupillary sign. It indicates severe midbrain damage usually from compression by a mass with raised intracranial pressure. Other causes are use of mydiatric drops, ingestion of anticholinergic drugs and direct ocular trauma. Occasionally in large cerebral haemorrhage that affects the thalamus, there may be unilateral meiosis. Bilaterally reactive small pupils (1-2.5mm) but not pinpoint are seen in metabolic encephalopathies. They may also be seen in bilateral deep hemispheric lesions like hydrocephalous or thalamic haemorrhage. Pinpoint pupils (1mm) are characteristics of pontine haemorrhage, narcotic or barbiturate overdose. These are differentiated by the response to naloxone and the eye movements.

Fundoscopy

Fundoscopy in an unconscious patient is also carried out in a dark room. You should use your right eye to examine the patient's right eye and vice versa. You should never go face on with the patient. It is possible to examine the optic disc and surrounding retina without dilatation of the pupil. The finding of swollen optic discs, or papilloedema, on ophthalmoscopy is a key sign, as this indicates raised intracranial pressure (ICP) which could be due to hydrocephalus, benign intracranial hypertension (aka pseudotumor cerebri) or brain tumor, amongst other conditions.

Eye movements

The spontaneous eye movements are observed by lifting the lids and noting the resting position and the spontaneous movements of the globes. Resistance to opening and the speed of closure reduces progressively as the coma deepens. *Beware of a supposedly unconscious patient that resists opening of eyes.* Note whether the eye movements are present. If they are present, then check whether they are conjugate or dysconjugate. Spontaneous eye movements in coma are usually horizontal roving with the eyes moving in parallel. This finding exonerates the midbrain and pons. Loss of this horizontal roving of the eye indicates damage to the pons on the opposite side of the lesion or the frontal lobe on the same side. It is said that *'the eyes look towards a hemispheric lesion and away from a brain stem lesion'*. In rare cases, the eyes may turn paradoxically away from the side of a deep hemispheric lesion (wrong-way eyes).

Note the prescence of ocular bobbing and ocular dipping.

In ocular bobbing, there is a brisk downward and slow upward movement of the eyes with loss of horizontal eye movement. It is diagnostic of bilateral pontine damage, usually from thrombosis of the basilar artery.

Ocular dipping is a slower arrhythmic downward movement followed by a faster upward movement in patients with normal reflex horizontal gaze. It indicates diffuse cortical anoxic damage.

Occulocephalic Reflexes/Dolls eye manouvre

If the patient is too drowsy to test voluntary eye movements, the occulocephalic reflexes are tested. Elicit these movements by moving the head from side to side or vertically. The vertical movements will be resisted in patients with meningeal irritation from meningitis or subarachnoid haemorrhage. The movements should not be carried out in persons with head or multiple traumas because of a possible concomitant cervical injury.

The usual response is the movement of the eyes in the opposite direction (like the dolls eye) hence the name. However, visual fixation suppresses these movements in the conscious person. The presence of these occulocephalic reflexes also signifies the integrity of the brain stem. The absence of the reflex on one side indicates an ipsilateral pontine lesion. Complete absence of the movements doll eye may be found in both extensive structural lesion of the brain stem and in deep metabolic coma. It is however intact in most patients with drug induced coma. Intact occulocephalic movements also indicate that the 3rd 4th and 6th cranial nerves are intact.

Oculovestibular response

These are also called thermal or caloric reflexes. The patient lies on the couch with head at 30°. Irrigate the external canal with water at 30° then at 44° for 30-40 seconds. Cold water induces nystagmus away from the ear been irrigated while warm water induces nystagmus towards the tested ear (COWS-cold water opposite, warm water same).

The absence of nystagmus despite conjugate deviation of the globes signifies that the cerebral hemispheres are damaged or depressed. Nystagmus cannot occur in the comatose patient because it requires ocular fixation. The loss of conjugate ocular movements indicates brain stem damage. It is important to inspect the tympanic membrane on each side before irrigating the external auditory meatus. This is because there may be a perforation.

8.46 Patterns of respiration

Alteration in the rhythm and pattern of respiration is an important aspect of the examination. The following patterns may be noted.

Agonal gasps

These reflect bilateral lower brainstem damage and are well known as the terminal respiratory pattern of severe brain damage.

Apneustic respiration
It is a pattern of breathing characterized by a prolonged inspiratory phase followed by expiratory apnoea. There is deep gasping sighing respiration with a pause at full inspiration. Thereafter, there is a brief insufficient relief. The rate of apneustic breathing is usually around 1.5 breaths per minute. Apneustic breathing is often associated with head injury.

Ataxic respiration
This is irregular, slow, deep, gasping respiration sometimes associated with hiccups. It occurs in progressive transtentorial herniation.

Biot's respiration
This is completely irregular. There is no pattern to it. The pattern of breathing is characterized by groups of quick, shallow inspirations followed by regular or irregular periods of apnoea. Causes include damage to the medulla due to strokes or trauma. It can also be caused by pressure on the medulla exerted by uncal or tentorial herniation. Opiod use is another cause. Biot's respiration generally indicates a poor prognosis

Cheyne-Stokes respiration
Cheyne –Stokes respiration is a cyclic form of respiration. There is a period of very rapid breaths followed by a phase of gradually deepening respiration and ends with an apnoeic spell for a few seconds (crescendo-decrescendo). The cycle is repeated. Cheyne-Stoke respiration in a comatose patient is a sign of large unilateral space occupying

lesion with brain stem deterioration. This can occur in subarachnoid haematoma. It can also be seen in bilateral brain lesions from other causes like cerebral infarction or meningitis. It commonly accompanies light coma.

Central pontine hyperventilation

In central pontine hyperventilation, there is a deep regular breathing. There may be interspersed deep sighs or yawns which precede the development of this respiratory pattern. It may occur with rostral brain damage.

Kussmaul respiration

This deep rapid sighing respiration usually implies metabolic acidosis. Metabolic ketoacidosis and uraemia are the commonest causes.

A similar pattern may occur in some patients with respiratory failure and hepatic coma. It may also occur with pontomesencephalic lesions. *Shallow, slow but regular respiration suggests metabolic or drug depression.*

Paradoxical respiration

In this type of respiration, all or part of the lung is deflated during inspiration and inflated during expiration: a paradox. It is seen in flail chest after trauma where there is fracture of ribs with a frozen section which does not connect with other parts of the thoracic cavity. It is also seen in diaphragmatic paralysis.

8.47 Cranial nerves examination in the unconscious patient

Cranial examination in the unconscious patient is difficult since the required patient's cooperation is not available. However, few cranial nerves can be examined in an unconscious patient as follows.

Optic nerve
This can be partially examined with the pupillary reflexes. The pupillary response also examines the oculomotor nerve to some extent. In patients who are drowsy, the visual field could be tested with visual menace or threat. This consists of threatening the left field of the face and thereafter, the right side. The fingers are usually used by the bedside. The normal response is a rapid eye closure; the blink is a protective reflex. Hemianopia is detected this way. It may also signify hemineglect.

Oculomotor, Trochlear and Abducens nerves
These can be examined to some extent by the eye movements. The doll eye movements are particularly important. These nerves have to be intact before the movements occur. Individual nerve palsies could be noted. Palsy of all three nerves in the prescence of proptosis indicates carvenous sinus thrombosis. It may also occur in nasopharyngeal tumours.

Facial nerve
The facial nerve is examined by applying bilateral supraorbital pain. Failure to grimace on one side indicates facial weakness on that side.

Vestibulocochlear Nerve
The occulovestibular/ caloric test described above is also a test for the vestibulocochlear nerve,

Motor examination
Observe the attitude and spontaneous movements of the limbs; note any asymmetric limb movement. The weaker limb is usually laterally rotated. A patient who is moving all the limbs actively does not have weakness of any limb. In patients who are not moving any limbs detection of weakness is done by comparing the response of the limbs to painful stimulus. The stimulus could be applied to the sternum. For the lower limbs, the stimulus is applied to the Achilles tendon. If pain produces an asymmetric response, then limb weakness is present. If the patient localizes with one arm, hold this down to ensure that a similar response cannot be elicited from the other limb.

The tendon reflexes may be asymmetrical. In most comatose patients, both plantar reflexes are extensor. Global power or power in indiv1idual muscle groups is usually not examined.

8.49 Sensory examination
This is difficult since patient's cooperation is needed. However pain sensation can be examined. The patient may respond to the painful stimulus. The absence of response on one side may indicate hemisensory loss.

8.48 Signs of Meningeal Irritation

Neck stiffness
Neck stiffness is the resistance to the flexion of the neck. *Resistance to neck extension or side-ways movement is not considered neck stiffness.* Passively flex the neck to check for neck stiffness. In meningeal irritation, neck flexion causes pain in the posterior part of the neck which may radiate to the back in which the unconscious patient may show a response. . The movement is also restricted by the extensor muscles of the neck. Neck stiffness in the unconscious patient is almost pathognomonic for meningitis but is also seen in subarachnoid haemorrhage. In extreme cases of neck stiffness, there may be neck retraction though this is rare; it was formerly a feature of untreated tuberculous meningitis particularly in children. The retraction could be so severe the child is severely bent backwards and looks like a tripod (tripod sign); in which case the retracted neck feels like a third limb.Neck stiffness is very sensitive in unconscious patients; having more reliability that Kernig's sign.

Kernig's sign
The Kernig's sign is elicited while the patient is in the supine position. Flex the thigh on the abdomen while the knee is already flexed; thereafter attempt to extend the knee. This attempt to passively extend the knee elicits pain and spasms of the hamstrings. The spasm of the hamstring muscle should be demonstrated by palpation.

Brudzinski's sign

The Brudzinski's sign is also elicited while the person is lying supine. Here, a passive flexion of the neck will lead to a spontaneous flexion of the hips and knees. In fact, it is wise to look out for the Brudzinski sign while examining for neck stiffness. Kernig's and Brudzinski's signs are not very sensitive especially in unconscious patients. They may also be absent or reduced in the extremes of life, in immune-compromised patients and in those with severely depressed mental status. *Neck stiffness is more sensitive.*

Other systems
The cardiovascular, respiratory and abdomen should also be fully examined in the evaluation of the unconscious patient.

8.5 Conclusion

In conclusion, a proper painstaking examination of the unconscious patient is extremely revealing. Extreme attention should be paid to supposedly minor details. The general examination is vital in guiding to more specific examinations of the nervous system.

FURTHER READING

1. Baliga R R: 250 short cases in clinical Medicine 3rd Ed Saunders 2001.
2. Epstein RJ. Medicine for examinations 4th Ed Canada 2006
3. Kasper DL, Fauci A S, Hauser S L, Longo D L, Jameson J L, Loscalzo J: Harrison's Principles of Internal Medicine; 19th Ed New York 2015
4. Lindsay K W. Bone I: Neurology and Neurosurgery Illustrated 4th Ed Edinburgh 2005
5. MoCA Version August 18, 2010
© Z. Nasreddine MD www.mocatest.org
6Rohkhamm R. Colour Atlas of Neurology 2ND Ed Stuttgart 2004
7. Ropper AH, Brown R H: Adams and Victor' Principles of Neurology 8th Ed New York 2005
8. Swash M, Glynn M: Hutchinson Clinical Methods 22nd Ed Edinburgh 2007
9. Walker HK, MD, Hall WD, MD, Hurst JW; Clinical Methods, the History, Physical, and Laboratory Examinations 3rd Ed Boston 1990

INDEX

Abadie's sign 115
Abdominal reflexes 101
Abducens nerve 69-71
Abnormal gaits 104-108
Abnormal movements 16-18
Absence seizures 11
Accesory nerve 82
Accommodation 66, 71
Address 4
Adie's tonic pupil 66, 127
Age 4
Aging gait 107
Agonal gasps 148
Agraphthesia 118
Alcohol history 25
Allen- Cleckley sign 102
Almond smell 138
Alternating anisocoria 127
Ammonia smell 138
Anhidrosis 128
Anisocoria 67, 145
Ankle clonus 99
Ankle Extensors 94
Ankle eversion 94
Ankle Flexors 94
Ankle inversion 94
Ankle jerk 99
Anomia 46
Anosmia 59
Antiphosholipid syndrome 23
Aphasia 44, 45
Apneustic Respiration 137, 149
Appearance 33, 127
Apraxic gait 104

Argyll-Robertson pupil 65
Arm Abduction Test 133
Arnold – Chiari 31
Ash leaf 31
Asymmetric limb response 37, 144
Asymmetric movement 83
Asymmetric tonic reflex 52
Astereognosis 120
Asterixis 57, 58
Atasia- abasia 105
Ataxic dysarthria 46
Ataxic respiration 149
Athetosis 17
Attention 47
Auditory memory 41
Automatic Walk Reflex 56
Autonomic nervous system 126-129
Babkin reflex 53
Ballismus 17
Barber chair phenomenon 134
Barbinski response 102
Barbinski rising sign 92
Battle sign 139
Beevor's sign 92
Benign Paroxysmal Positional Vertigo 19
Behaviour 33
Bell's palsy 33
Bell's Phenomenon 75
Biceps 90
Biceps jerk 97
Biernacki sign 115
Bing's Sign 102
Biodata 3-7
Biot's respiration 149
Bjerrum screen 63, 64
Blink 34, 143

BPPV 19, 78
Bracelet 136
Brachial di 88
Brachioradialis 90, 91
Brachioradialis jerk 97
Bradykinesia 31
Bradyphrenia 48
Brainstem reflex 36 144
Broca's aphasia 43
Brudzinski sign 122, 154
Bruising 139
Bulk of muscles 83-84
Bull neck 31
Cafe au lait 31
Caloric Test 79
Carpal tunnel syndrome 133,134
Cautious gait 109
Central Pontine hyperventilation 150
Central Scotoma 64
Central vertigo 19
Cerebellar ataxic gait 105
Cerebellar function 122-125
Cervical spine 130
Chaddock sign 102
Chaddock reflex 102
Cheyene- Stokes 136,149
Chorda tympani 74
Chorea 17, 85
Choriocarcinoma 24
Chunking 38
Clasp knife rigidity 86
Cogwheel rigidity 86
Colour Vision 60, 64
Coma 16,136-154
Communication 33
Comprehension 44

Complex partial seizures 11
Comprehension 44
Concentration 45
Conductive deafness 77
Confrontation tests 62
Confusion 16
Conjugate movement 72
Consciousness 15, 33, 142
Corneal reflex 72, 100
Cornell reflex 102
Cortical sensation 118-120
Counting test 131
COWS 79,148
CRANIAL NERVES 59-81
Cremasteric reflex 101
Crescendo-decrescendo 147
Crossed Adductor Reflex 53
Crossed Extension Reflex 53
Curtain test 132
Dance Reflex 56
Decerebrate posture 36, 141
Decibels 77
Declarative memory 41, 42
Decorticate posture 141
Deep tendon reflexes 95-98
Dental gap 31
Diabetic neuropathy 114
Diaphragm 92
Digit span 42
Difficulty in speaking 22
Disorientation 40
Distal Symmetrical poly neuropathy 114
Distant Vision 62
Dix-Hallpike 77
Dizziness 19
Doll eye manoeuvre 147

Dorsal midbrain palsy 67
Dorsi flexors 94
Drug History 24
Drunken Sailor gait 105
DSPN 113,115
Dysarthria 44-46
Dysdiadokinesia 124
Dysmetria 123,124
Dysmorphic features 31
Dysphasia 42- 45
Dysphonia 46
Dystonia 17, 85
Dystonic gait 105
Echymoses 138
Elbow clonus 99
Elbow extension 90
Elbow flexion 90
Embrace Reflex 55
Entrapment Neuropathies 19
Epicriptic sensory 110
Episodic memory 41
Erector spinae 85
Ethnic Group 5, 6
Explicit Memory 40
Expressive aphasia 43
External Auditory meatus 77
Extensor plantar response 102
Eye movements 146
Eye Opening 37
Facial Asymmetry 31
Facial atrophy 76
Facial nerve 73-75
Family and Social history 24
Fencing Posture 52
Festinant gait 106
Fetor hepaticus 138

Fever 137
Fibromas 31
Finger abduction 91
Finger extension 91
Finger Extension Reflex 59
Finger flexion 91
Finger Flexion reflex 98
Finger-nose test 123
Fishy smell 138
Fistula Test 78
Flaccid dysarthria 46
Flappy tremors 57
Flexor plantar response 102
Fluent aphasia 44
Foot drop 106
Forearm pronation 90
Forearm supination 90
Forgetfulness 20
Free-field tests 77
Frontal lobe gait 104
Fundoscopy 62, 68, 146
Gag Reflex 79
Gallant Reflex 54
GCS 34
General Examination 30
Gingival hypertrophy 31
Glabella Tap Reflex 54
Gladiator gait 106
Glasgow Coma Scale 34, 142
Glossopharyngeal nerve 79
Glove and stocking 114
Goldman perimeter 67
Gonda Allen sign 102
Gordon sign 102
Graphethesia 118
Guillain Barre 14

Gustatory sweating 128
Guyon canal syndrome 133
Hallpike Manouvre 79
Hand grip 91
Haneal sign 114
Headache   8-11
Heel shin test 124
Hemianopia 67
Hemi 88
Hemiballismus 17
Hemichorea 17
Hemineglect 44
Hemiparesis 88
Hemipegia 88
Hemiplegic gait 106
Herpes Zoster Ophthalmicus 31
High Steppage gait 107
Hip abductors 93
Hip adductors 93
Hip extensors 93
Hip flexors 93
History Taking   8-26
Hoffman's reflex 98
Holmes –Adie syndrome 66
Hoover's sign 92
Horner's syndrome 69, 128, 144
Humphrey field analyser 67
Hyperacuisis 75
Hyperkinetic dysarthria 46
Hypermetria 124
Hyper nasality 47
Hyperpyrexia 138
Hyperthermia 138
Hypertonia 85
Hypoglossal nerve 80
Hypometria 124

Hypothermia 137
Hypotonia 85
Hypotonic dysarthria 46
Hysterical gait 105
Ice pack test 132
Immediate memory 38
Implicit memory 41
Increasing pallor 138
Inferior Obliques 71
Inferior recti 71
Informant   2, 26
Infranuclear 75, 76
Insight 48
Intelligence 47
Inverse Supinator jerk 97
Isihara chart 66
Jacksonian March 11, 18
Jaeger card 63
Jaw jerk 72, 97
Judgment 48
Kernig's sign 122, 153
Knee Extensors 93
Knee Flexors 94
Knee jerk 98
Kussmaul respiration 152
Jendrassik manoeuvre 97
Judgment 50
Lateral maleolar sign 102
Lateral Pterygoid 73
Latismus Dorsi 91
Laundau Reflex 55
Lacunar stroke 18
Lead pipe rigidity 86
Lhermitte's sign 134
Light-Near dissociation 67
Light Reflex 64,144

Light touch 114
Liver flap 60
Long term memory 39
Loss of Consciousness 15, 16
Lumbar spine 131
Marche a petit pas 107
Marcus Gunn pupil 66
Marital Status 5
Masseter muscle 73
MCI 50
Medial Longitudunal Fasciculus 66
Medical Research Council 87
Memory 20 37-42
Memory Loss 20
Meniere's disease 19
Meningeal irritation 121-123, 153
Meningococaaemia 31, 137
Mild cognitive impairment 50
Minimental State Examination (MMSE) 49
MMSE 49
Mo CA 50-51
Moniz sign 103
Mono 88
Monolalia 48
Monoloudness 48
Monopitch 48
Montreal Cognitive Assessment 50-51
Moro's reflex 55
Motor Neurone Disease 81
Motor Response 35
Multifocal myoclonic jerks 140
Muscular Dystrophy 85
Muscle Myokimia 85
Muscles of the trunk 92
Myasthenia gravis 131-133
Myasthenic weakness 14

Mydiatric 65, 66
Myerson sign 54
Myoclonic jerks 85, 141
Myoclonus 17
Myopathic gait 107
Name   3
Naming 44
Naso-labial folds 75
Near Response 68
Near Vision 63
Neck flexors 93
Neck stiffness 121, 153
Negative symptoms 18
Neurocutaeneous 31
Neurofibromatosis 31
Neuromas 31
Neurosyphilis 67
Noiceptive sensory 110
Non fluent aphasia 45
Non positional vertigo 78
Noonan's syndrome 31
Numbness 18
Nystagmus 71
Obstetrics and Gynaecology history 23
Occulocephalic movements 147
Occulomotor nerve 68-71
Occulovestibular response 148
Occupation 6
Olfactory nerve 59, 60
Oppenheim reflex 103
Optic nerve 60-69
Orbicularis Oculi 75
Ordours 138
Orthostatic Hypotension 129
Orientation 36
Oschner's clasp test 134

Pain sensation 113
Palatal reflex 72, 100
Palmar Avoidance reflex 55
Palmar grasp Reflex 55
Palmo-Mental Reflex 55
Papilloedema 146
Para 88
Paracentral Scotoma 65
Parachute Reflex 56
Paradoxical Respiration 152
Paraparetic gait 108
Paresis 88
Parietal drift 86
Parinaud's Syndrome 66
Parkinson Disease 17, 18, 85, 106
Parkinsonian gait 106
Parosmia 61, 62
Past Medical History 22, 23
Patellar clonus 99
Patterns of Limb weakness 95-96
Pectoralis major 90
Perimetry 63
Peripheral vertigo 19
Perisylvian Apasia 44
PERRLA 61, 127
Petechial haemorrhage 138
Phalen's manoeuvre 134
Pharyngeal reflex 79
Pinpoint pupil 145
Pins and needles 18
Pitre's sign 114
Placing Reflex 55
Plantar flexors 94
Plantar reflex 101-103
Platysma 75
Plegia 88

Plexopathies 19
Point's Cardineaux 55
Pointing test 134
Positional vertigo 78
Positive symptoms 18
Postural Hypotension 129
Posture 140
Potts disease 14
Pout Reflex 56
Power of muscles 87
Pregnancy and birth history 24
Presenting complaint 8
Pressure 114
Primitive Reflexes 52-57
Procedural Memory 41
Progressive multifocal leuco encephalopathy 23
Pronator drift 86
Proprioception 116
Proprioceptive sense 116-117
Proptosis 33
Proximal Myopathy 92
Pseudo- Isochromatic Plates 65
Ptosis 65
Pupillary Light Reflexes 64, 126, 144
Quadri 88
Quadriplegia 88
Race 6
Raccoon eyes 139
Reading 45
Recent Memory 43
Receptive aphasia 44
Recurrent abortions 23
Red glass test 70
Red pin confrontation 63
Repetition 44
Religion 5

Rhomberg's test 78,125
Rigidity 86
Rinne negative 76
Rinne positive 76
Rinne's test 76
Role of Informants 26
Rooting Reflex 55
Rostral Interstitial nucleus 67
Saddle area 111
Scanning Speech 46
Scapular reflex 100
Schafer sign 103
Scissors gait 108
Scotoma 70
Search Reflex 55
Seborrhoea 31
Secondary memory 38
Seizures 11-13
Semantic Memory 40
Semi coma 34
Sensorineural deafness 78
Sensory dermatomes 111-112
Sensory disturbances 18
Sensory inattention 119
Sensory modalities 112
Sensory seizure 18
Serial 3 Test 47
Serial 7 Test 47
Serratus Anterior 89
Shagreen patches 31
Short term memory 38
Shoulder abduction 89
Shoulder adduction 89
Simultagnosia 44
Significant Headaches 10-11
Slapping gait 106

SLE 23
Sleep test 132
Smoking 26
Snarl 31
Snarl test 132
Snellen chart 61
Snout Reflex 56
SOCRATES 8-10
Spastic dysarthria 45
Speech 44-47
Spine 129-131
Spine extensors 92
Staccato Speech 46
Stamping gait 107
Stapedius 74
Startle Reflex 55
Stelwag Sign 31
Stepping Reflex 56
Sternocleidomastoid 81
Stereognosis 119
Stransky sign 103
Strength of muscles 87
Strumpell sign 103
Stupor 34
Sucking Reflex 57
Sunset eyes 66
Supinator jerk 97
Superficial reflexes 100-104
Supra nuclear 75, 77
Supra orbital 37
Sustained clonus 99
Stepping Reflex 56
Superficial abdominal reflex 100
Superior Obliques 69
Superior Recti 69
Supraspinatus 90

Swallowing Reflex 75
Sweating abnormalities 127,128
Swinging Light Reflex 66
Systemic Lupus Erythematosus 23
Tabes Dorsalis 66
Tactile sensibility 114
Tandem walk 125
Tangent Screen 66
Teasdale and Jennett 34
Temperature sensation 114
Tetra 88
Tinel's sign 133
Teres Major 90
Thermal Reflexes 148
Thomas sign 103
Thoracic spine 131
Throckmorton sign 104
Thumb extension 91
Thumb Opposition 91
Thyrotoxicosis 33
Tics 17
Titubation 18
Todd's palsy 11
Toe extensors 95
Toe flexors 95
Tone of muscles 84-85
Toppling gait 108
Tournique's test 134
Tracheotomy tube 37, 143
Trail making test 47
Transcortical Aphasia 46
Transient loss of consciousness 15
Trapezius 90
Tredlenburg gait 108
Tremors 17
Tri 88

Triceps 90
Triceps jerk 98
Trigeminal nerve 71-73
Trigeminal reflexes 73, 74
Tripod sign 153
Trismus 31
Trochlear nerve 68-71
Turner's syndrome 31
Truncal Incurvation 54
Tuberous Sclerosis 31
Two point discrimination 118
Unconsciousness 15, 16, 136-153
Upward gaze palsy 72
Unterberger test 78
Vagus nerve 79
Ventral Suspension Reflex 54
Verbal Response 35
Vertical gaze palsy 66
Vertigo 19
Vestibular gait 109
Vestibular Migraine 19
Vestibulocochlear nerve 75-77
Vibration sense 116
Visual acuity 61, 63
Visual Fields 61-63
Visual memory 44
von Frey hair 116
Waddling gait 107
Walking 124, 125
Weakness 13-15
Weber's Test 76
Wernicke's aphasia 50
Wernicke –Korsakoff 25
Wrist extensors 91
Wrist flexors 91
Writing 47

Wrong way eyes 146

Bertha C Ekeh

Clinical Neurology Made Easy

www.ingramcontent.com/pod-product-compliance
Lightning Source LLC
Chambersburg PA
CBHW031626210526
45464CB00004B/1766